# Basic
# Math for Nursing and Allied Health

## Lynn M. Egler, BS (Health Science), RMA, AHI, CPhT

*Author, Consultant*
*LME Solutions*
*Saint Clair Shores, Michigan*

*Adjunct Faculty*
*Baker College*
*Clinton Township, Michigan*

## Denise J. Propes, CPhT

*Senior and Lead Pharmacy Technician*
*Research Pharmacy*
*University of Michigan Health System*
*Ann Arbor, Michigan*

## Alice J. Brown, RN

*Registered Nurse/Trauma Nurse*
*Emergency Department*
*Virginia Beach General Hospital*
*Virginia Beach, Virginia*

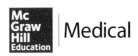
Mc Graw Hill Education | Medical

New York   Chicago   San Francisco   Athens   London   Madrid
Mexico City   Milan   New Delhi   Singapore   Sydney   Toronto

**Basic Math for Nursing and Allied Health**

1 2 3 4 5 6 7 8 9 0   CTP/CTP   19 18 17 16 15 14

ISBN 978-0-07-182907-6
MHID 0-07-182907-5

---

### Notice

Medicine is an ever-changing science. As new research and clinical experience broaden our knowledge, changes in treatment and drug therapy are required. The authors and the publisher of this work have checked with sources believed to be reliable in their efforts to provide information that is complete and generally in accord with the standards accepted at the time of publication. However, in view of the possibility of human error or changes in medical sciences, neither the authors nor the publisher nor any other party who has been involved in the preparation or publication of this work warrants that the information contained herein is in every respect accurate or complete, and they disclaim all responsibility for any errors or omissions or for the results obtained from use of the information contained in this work. Readers are encouraged to confirm the information contained herein with other sources. For example and in particular, readers are advised to check the product information sheet included in the package of each drug they plan to administer to be certain that the information contained in this work is accurate and that changes have not been made in the recommended dose or in the contraindications for administration. This recommendation is of particular importance in connection with new or infrequently used drugs.

---

This book was set in Minion Pro by Thomson Digital.
The editors were Michael Weitz and Cindy Yoo.
The production supervisor was Richard Ruzycka.
Project management was provided by Saloni Narang, Thomson Digital.
The designer was Elise Lansdon; the cover designer was Thomas DePierro.
China Translation & Printing Services, Ltd. was printer and binder.

This book is printed on acid-free paper.

**Library of Congress Cataloging-in-Publication Data**

Egler, Lynn M., author.
 Basic math for nursing and allied health / Lynn M. Egler, Denise J. Propes.
  pages ; cm
 Includes bibliographical references and index.
 ISBN-13: 978-0-07-182907-6 (paperback : alk. paper)
 ISBN-10: 0-07-182907-5 (paperback : alk. paper) 1. Mathematics—Textbooks. 2. Fractions—Textbooks. I. Propes, Denise J., author. II. Title.
 [DNLM: 1. Mathematics—Nurses' Instruction. 2. Mathematics—Problems and Exercises. QA107.2]
 QA107.2.E35 2014
 513.2'1—dc23

2014000033

Recipes presented in exercises are for educational purposes only.

McGraw-Hill Education books are available at special quantity discounts to use as premiums and sales promotions, or for use in corporate training programs. To contact a representative, please visit the Contact Us pages at www.mhprofessional.com.

OCT 2 0 2014

# Acknowledgments

**Contributor**  Kelly Washington, MLA, Adjunct Professor, Kaplan University, Chicago, Illinois.

**Reviewer**  Jennifer L. Jiminey, Medical Assistant/Medical Office Manager, Tete Oniango, MD, PLLC.

**Information Technology and Administrative Support**  James Propes

A special thank-you to Michael Weitz, Laura Libretti, Cindy Yoo, and all of the McGraw-Hill staff that helped develop and design this project.

# Authors Biography

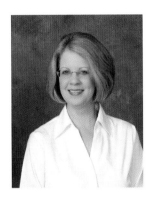

**Lynn M. Egler, BS (Health Science), RMA, AHI, CPhT,** has worked in the health care and education fields across the country for the past 30 years. She served in the United States Navy as a Hospital Corpsman and Emergency Medical Technician during Operations Desert Shield and Desert Storm. Mrs. Egler's health care experience also includes emergency department, endoscopy, anesthesia and recover, hospital pediatrics and maternal health, hospital laboratory, family practice, and retail pharmacy.

As a dedicated educator, she has held the positions of Medical Programs Coordinator, Medical Assistant and Medical Office Specialist Program Director, Medical Assistant Education Chair, Allied Health Instructor, Externship Coordinator, American Heart Association CPR Instructor and Training Center Faculty, and Curriculum Content Specialist for college accreditation visits with the Accreditation Counsel for Continuing Education and Training (ACCET). Mrs. Egler has developed and standardized multiple curricula for thirteen college campuses across five states, including medical assisting, medical office administration, dental assisting, surgical technician, and pharmacy technician programs. She has authored educational materials and textbooks with McGraw-Hill Higher Education and McGraw-Hill Professional.

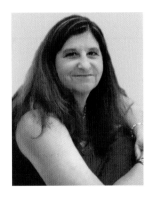

**Denise J. Propes, CPhT,** has actively worked in the pharmacy profession for 30 years. She spent many years as a pharmacy technician in various retail settings before moving on to a hospital pharmacy environment. Ms. Propes is an active member of multiple pharmacy and health care organizations and associations. Ms. Propes has authored and presented educational materials at national pharmacy conferences. She has held the positions of Allied Health Instructor and Pharmacy Technician Instructor. Ms. Propes has taught medical terminology, allied health math, and pharmacy technician courses at institutions throughout Michigan. Ms. Propes has assisted in implementing and instructing the pharmacy operations laboratory section of a health-system pharmacy course at the University of Michigan College of Pharmacy for the past 3 years. She has reviewed and updated pharmacy educational documents for several organizations and companies, and has co-authored textbooks for McGraw Hill Professional. Ms. Propes is currently employed at the University of Michigan Medical Center as the Lead Pharmacy Technician in the Research Pharmacy. She also teaches Pharmacy Technician education classes for the Lenawee Intermediate School District (LISD) Technical Center Adult Learning Services Program.

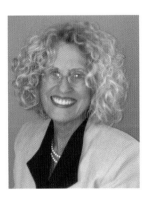

**Alice J. Brown, RN,** has been a Registered Nurse for over 30 years. She began her nursing career in New Jersey. As a military spouse, Alice J. Brown has worked in several states as well as a US territory. She has extensive experience in emergency and trauma nursing. Alice J. Brown's additional areas of experience include cardiac care, intensive care, orthopedics, oncology, outpatient surgery, and gastroenterology. She has also practiced as a Medical Officer on Holland America cruise lines.

# Contents

# Preface

Nursing and Allied Health professionals not only need to be knowledgeable in their specialized professions, they also need to be proficient and confident in their basic math skills in order to master dosage calculations and complex formulas used in their professions daily. It is imperative that Nursing and Allied Health professionals have a solid math skill base, and comprehend the importance of how accurately performing dosage calculations, and complex specialized formulas, directly affects patient care and outcomes. *Basic Math for Nursing and Allied Health* is written in an easy-to-understand format that takes the fear out of performing basic math skills, and is designed to walk students through the step-by-step processes needed to master basic math skills.

*Basic Math for Nursing and Allied Health* uses a math-friendly approach of connecting basic math concepts with everyday activities, enabling the student to advance and master the more complex calculations and formulas used by Nursing and Allied Health professionals. This textbook walks students through multiple basic math concepts from Arabic and Roman numerals, addition, subtraction, multiplication, division, fractions, decimals, percentages, ratios and proportions, to conversion factors between household and metric measurements. A unique feature of this text is the chapter case studies, which not only show the mathematical concepts related to the everyday practices of making recipes, shopping sales, calculating costs, and adding correct totals, but also show the students how to effectively use case studies to master the art of interpreting story problems. Students learn to extract the correct information needed to properly set up and solve the mathematical equations associated with each case study. In today's advanced technological society many rely on the use of calculators to perform everyday math problems. This text has a "Manual Math" feature box to reinforce the student's confidence and knowledge in mastering basic math skills. As students work through each chapter, they will master the basic math skills needed to gain the proficiency and confidence needed to advance to mastering the more complex calculations and formulas performed by Nursing and Allied Health professionals.

## FEATURES

*Basic Math for Nursing and Allied Health* will include the following features to reinforce student learning:

- "Recipes for Success" Case Study scenarios with story problem extraction and equation set-up and solving exercises.

- "Manual Math" tips and reminder boxes

- Key terms

- Learning outcomes

- Chapter openers explaining the importance of the chapter

- Practice equations after each concept presented

- Chapter summary

- End-of-chapter practice tests

- Comprehensive review and exam

# 1 Understanding Numbers, Story Problems, and Numbering Systems

## INTRODUCTION

Reading for numbers and information in story problems and understanding story problems and numbering systems are very important skills healthcare professionals use in everyday practices. Whether you are a medical assistant, pharmacy technician, dental assistant, nurse, or patient care technician, you will need to be able to read, interpret, identify, extract, convert, and solve problems using numbers. This is all achievable by using basic reading and math skills and understanding numbering systems. We use basic math skills every day. Many of us probably don't even realize how many times in a day we use math. Chapter 1 will walk you through the steps of reading for numbers and the information used in story problems. You will learn how to identify and extract the information needed to set up proper equations, which you will use to master the skill of solving story problems. You will also learn Arabic numbers and Roman numerals, and how to convert between the two very different numbering systems.

## LEARNING OBJECTIVES

1. Identify information needed to solve story problems.
2. Extract pertinent information from story problems needed to set up proper equations.
3. Perform basic math skills to solve story problems.
4. Understand Arabic numbers and Roman numeral systems.
5. Understand Arabic numbers combined in different ways have different values.
6. Recognize Roman numerals and Arabic numbers.
7. Convert Roman numerals to Arabic numbers.
8. Express Arabic numbers as Roman numerals.

## READING FOR NUMBERS

Reading for numbers and properly interpreting them is a critical part of being an allied health professional or nurse. You are the numbers detective hired by your medical employer to solve many number mysteries presented daily in allied health settings. Numbers are written in many different ways, which can change the value of the numbers. When reading for numbers, it is important to understand the value of the number you are reading. If the value of a number is interpreted incorrectly, errors can occur that can negatively affect patient outcomes, such as a medication dosage error.

Numbers can be written using words, letters, digits, and symbols. We write personal checks using words, digits, and symbols. Numbers are also written in different values such as whole numbers, fractions, decimals, and percentages. Let's look at the different ways to write the value of a one-dollar bill and a half dollar.

### EXAMPLE 1

The value of a one-dollar bill can be written as:

One dollar, a dollar, $1.00, 1.00, and 100% of a dollar.

**EXAMPLE   2**

The value of a half dollar:

   One-half dollar, a half dollar, ½ dollar, 50 cents, $0.50, .50, and 50% of a dollar.

   Now that you have an idea about the different ways numbers can be written, we will read the sentence below for numbers and write them in different ways.

   The local grocery store has eggs of sale for a $1.39 a dozen.

**EXAMPLE**

Eggs are on sale for $1.39 a dozen. $1.39 can be written as:

   $1.39, One dollar and 39 cents, 1.39

And a dozen eggs can be written as:

   A dozen eggs, One dozen eggs, 1 dozen eggs.

This can bring us to another question:

   How many eggs are in a dozen? There are 12 eggs in a dozen.

   Now we can add to the way we can write the value of a dozen eggs.

**EXAMPLE**

A dozen eggs can be written as:

   A dozen eggs, one dozen eggs, 1 dozen eggs, twelve eggs, and 12 eggs.

**Practice Exercise 1-1**   Read the following sentences for numbers and write the numbers using words, digits, letters, and symbols.

   **1.** A case of purple latex-free gloves costs $75.00

   A case         _____

   $75.00        _____

   **2.** There are 10 thin cardboard boxes of gloves in a full case.

   10 boxes      _____

   A full case   _____

   **3.** There are 50 gloves in each box of gloves.

   50 gloves     _____

   Each box      _____

Now that you have an idea about the different ways numbers can be written, we can add numbers to sentences and paragraphs to begin our detective work. The first step is to identify the number in the sentence and then determine the value. If you are reading a medical supply company sales ad and they have a case of purple latex-free gloves on sale for $75.00 a case, you need to determine if the sale price is a good value for your office. Based on the sentences in Practice Exercise 1.1, we know that 1 case of latex-free gloves is on sale for $75.00, each case has 10 thin cardboard boxes of gloves, and each thin cardboard box has 50 purple gloves.

# STORY PROBLEMS

Story problems, like basic math skills, are questions or problems we solve every day, many times without realizing it. Reading the story carefully and identifying and extracting information needed to solve the problem is the key. Reading story problems builds on the process used in reading for numbers. The story may not be asking for numbers, but you use the same idea of reading for the answer. The questions asked after a story problem are the problems you are trying to solve using the story. Story problems really aren't problems so to speak; they are simply questions that can be answered by reading a story. In working with story problems, it is always best to know what you are reading for, so read the questions (problems) that follow the story, before reading the actual story.

### EXAMPLE

*Using the medical supply company glove sale story, use the following questions to "read for" in the story.*

**Questions:**

What color are the gloves?

What type of glove is on sale?

What type of material are the boxes made of?

**Story:**

You are reading a medical supply company sales ad, and they have a case of purple latex-free gloves on sale for $75.00 a case. You need to determine if the sale price is a good value for your office. Each case contains 10 thin cardboard boxes of gloves, and each box contains 50 purple latex-free gloves.

In knowing what to read for, we can easily solve story problems. We now know from reading the medical supply company sale ad that the gloves are purple, latex-free, and are packed in thin cardboard boxes.

## Identifying and Extracting Information

To successfully solve story problems, information related to the questions being asked must be properly identified and extracted from the story. This is a skill required of allied health professionals, and one you can perfect.

Story problems many times include information that is not applicable to the question being asked. This can appear to be extraneous, or extra, information for the purpose of identifying the information needed for the question at hand; however, some extraneous information may pertain to future questions. Using the same medical supply sale scenario, we will identify and extract information needed to solve our problems as well as identify extraneous information.

### EXAMPLE

*Using the medical supply company glove sales story, use the following questions to "read for" in the story.*

**Questions:**

How much is a case of gloves on sale for?

How many boxes of gloves are in each case?

How many gloves are in each box of gloves?

*—Continued next page*

*Continued—*

### Story:

You are reading a medical supply company sales ad, and they have a case of purple latex-free gloves on sale for $75.00 a case. You need to determine if the sale price is a good value for your office. Each case contains 10 thin cardboard boxes of gloves, and each box contains 50 purple gloves.

Based on knowing what questions to read for, we know that 1 case of latex-free gloves is on sale for $75.00, each case has 10 thin cardboard boxes of gloves, and each thin cardboard box has 50 purple gloves.

### Extraneous Information:

Using the questions to read for in the story problem can help us identify extraneous (extra) information, not needed to solve the questions asked. The extraneous information is highlighted in the following sentences.

One case of latex-free gloves is on sale for $75.00.

Each case has 10 thin cardboard boxes of gloves.

Each box has 50 purple gloves.

The highlighted information in each sentence was not needed to answer the original question, thus being extraneous information for this set of questions or problems, but can pertain to other questions.

---

**Practice Exercise 1-2**   Using the medical supply company glove sale as our story, solve the problems and identify any extraneous information.

### Story Problem:

You are reading a medical supply company sales ad, and they have a case of purple latex-free gloves on sale for $75.00 a case. You need to determine if the sale price is a good value for your office. Each case contains 10 thin cardboard boxes of gloves, and each box contains 50 purple latex-free gloves.

What color are the gloves?

What type of glove is on sale?

What type of material are the boxes made of?

1. Identify any extraneous information, not needed to answer the story problem questions above, in the sentences below.

    One case of latex-free gloves is on sale for $75.00. _____

    Each case has 10 thin cardboard boxes of gloves. _____

    Each thin cardboard box has 50 purple gloves. _____

2. Now that you have read the questions and story, and have identified any extraneous information, solve the following story problem questions.

    What color are the gloves? _____

    What type of glove is on sale? _____

    What type of material are the boxes made of? _____

## Setting Up and Solving Equations

In reading story problems, not only is it important to be able to identify and extract information needed to solve the problems, it is equally as important to be able to set up and solve mathematical equations. The key to setting up and solving equations is to properly interpret what the story problem is asking. First, read the questions, next read the story, then interpret what is being asked, identify any extraneous information, identify and extract information, set up the equation, and then solve the equation to solve the story problem. In using the information learned in the previous two sections, and building on it, setting up and solving equations can be done by following the eight-step process shown in Table 1-1.

**TABLE 1-1  Steps to Setting up and Solving Equations for Story Problems**

| | |
|---|---|
| Step 1: | Read the questions |
| Step 2: | Read the story |
| Step 3: | Interpret what is being asked |
| Step 4: | Identify extraneous information |
| Step 5: | Identify and extract information needed to set up the equation |
| Step 6: | Set up the equation |
| Step 7: | Solve the equation |
| Step 8: | Solve the story problem |

## EXAMPLE

*Use the medical supply glove sale story to solve the following story problem:*

You are reading a medical supply company sales ad, and they have a case of purple latex-free gloves on sale for $75.00 a case. You need to determine if the sale price is a good value for your office. Each case contains 10 thin cardboard boxes of gloves, and each box contains 50 purple latex-free gloves.

How much would each box of gloves in the case cost? _____

**STEP 1** *Read the question.*

How much would each box of gloves in the case cost?

**STEP 2** *Read the story.*

You are reading a medical supply company sales ad, and they have a case of purple latex-free gloves on sale for $75.00 a case. You need to determine if the sale price is a good value for your office. Each case contains 10 thin cardboard boxes of gloves, and each box contains 50 purple latex-free gloves.

**STEP 3** *Interpret the question.*

The question is asking how much each box of gloves in the case costs. To get the cost per box, we need to divide the <u>price of the case</u> by the <u>number of boxes</u> in the case.

**STEP 4** *Identify extraneous information.*

*Each case costs $75.00.*

*Each case contains 10 thin cardboard boxes of gloves.*

*Each box contains 50 purple latex-free gloves.*

**STEP 5** *Identify and extract information needed to set up the equation.*

*Each case costs $75.00.*

*Each case contains 10 thin cardboard boxes of gloves.*

*Each box contains 50 purple latex-free gloves.*

Each case costs $75.00 and there are 10 boxes in a case.

*—Continued next page*

*Continued—*

**STEP 6**  *Set up the equation.*

Each case costs $75.00 and there are 10 boxes in a case.

$75.00 *case* ÷ 10 *boxes* =

**STEP 7**  *Solve the equation.*

$75.00 ÷ 10 *boxes* = $7.50 *per box*

**STEP 8**  *Solve the story problem.*

You are reading a medical supply company sales ad, and they have a case of purple latex-free gloves on sale for $75.00 a case. You need to determine if the sale price is a good value for your office. Each case contains 10 thin cardboard boxes of gloves, and each box contains 50 purple latex-free gloves.

How much would each box of gloves in the case cost?

*Solution to the story problem:*

Each box of gloves in the case would cost $7.50.

## Practice Exercise 1-3   Using the 7-step process in Table 1-1, solve the following story problem:

You are reading a medical supply company sales ad, and they have a case of purple latex-free gloves on sale for $75.00 a case. You need to determine if the sale price is a good value for your office. Each case contains 10 thin cardboard boxes of gloves, and each box contains 50 purple latex-free gloves.

How much would each glove cost?  _____

**STEP 1**  *Read the question.*

How much would each glove cost?

**STEP 2**  *Read the story.*

You are reading a medical supply company sales ad, and they have a case of purple latex-free gloves on sale for $75.00 a case. You need to determine if the sale price is a good value for your office. Each case contains 10 thin cardboard boxes of gloves. Each box of gloves costs $7.50, and each box contains 50 purple latex-free gloves.

**STEP 3**  *Interpret the question.*

The question is asking how much each glove in the case costs. To get the cost per glove, what do you need to do?

**STEP 4**  *Identify extraneous information.*

Each case of gloves costs $75.00.

Each case contains 10 thin cardboard boxes of gloves.

Each box of gloves costs $7.50.

Each box contains 50 purple latex-free gloves.

**STEP 5**  *Identify and extract information needed to set up the equation.*

Each case of gloves costs $75.00.

Each case contains 10 thin cardboard boxes of gloves.

Each box of gloves costs $7.50.

Each box contains 50 purple latex-free gloves.

**STEP 6** *Set up the equation*

_____ ÷ _____ =

**STEP 7** *Solve the equation*

_____ ÷ _____ =

**STEP 8** *Solve the story problem.*

You are reading a medical supply company sales ad, and they have a case of purple latex-free gloves on sale for $75.00 a case. You need to determine if the sale price is a good value for your office. Each box of gloves costs $7.50, and each box contains 50 purple latex-free gloves.

How much would each glove cost?

*Solution to the story problem:*

Each glove would cost _____.

# ARABIC NUMBERS

The Arabic number system is the number system that we use every day. The system consists of the ten digits **0**, **1**, **2**, **3**, **4**, **5**, **6**, **7**, **8**, and **9**, which can be combined in many ways to represent different number values and expressions. As an allied health professional or a nurse, it is important to understand our number system as well as the Roman numeral system as they are both commonly used in physician's orders.

## Number Values

**Arabic number *digits* combined in different ways have VERY different values.** Identifying and writing the digits correctly can have a direct impact on patient care. For example, a dose of **0.5 teaspoons** of a medication has a very different value than **5 teaspoons** of the same medication. Reading and writing numbers incorrectly can result in a medical error that may cause serious harm, or even death, to a patient.

> **EXAMPLE**
>
> **47 is a whole number**
>
> **4/7 is a fraction**
>
> **.47 is a decimal**

## Combining and Counting

Combining and counting using Arabic numbers is how we perform basic math. We have learned to count by using the following ten digits: 0, 1, 2, 3, 4, 5, 6, 7, 8, and 9. And the results are numbers formed by combining the digits.

> **EXAMPLE**
>
> Counting by 1: 1, 2, 3, 4, 5, 6, 7, 8, 9, 10, 11, 12, 13, 14, 15.
>
> In the list of numbers counting from 1 to 15, 1 through 9 are listed using a single digit, whereas 10 through 15 are listed by combining 2 digits.
>
> Counting by 10: 10, 20, 30, 40, 50, 60, 70, 80, 90, 100.
>
> In the list counting by 10, we combined 2 digits for 10 through 90, and three digits for 100.

Can we combine two numbers? Sure we can, let's combine the two digits of 15, with the 3 digits of 100. Together, 15 and 100 combined will produce the new number of 15100. **Combining digits is not the same as performing addition.** If we add 15 and 100, we would get the sum of 115.

> ### EXAMPLE
>
> 15 *and* 100 *combined is* 15100, **whereas** 15 + 100 = 115
>
> 15100 *has a much larger value than* 115.

As stated previously, the way numbers are written shows very different values. As an allied health professional or nurse you will learn to always pay close attention to the value of all the numbers that you work with because the patient's well-being depends on it.

**Practice Exercise 1-4**   Fill in the missing numbers in the following counting lines; then combine the digits of the numbers and add the numbers.

1. Counting by 2: 2, 4, _____, 8, 10, 12, _____, 16, 18, _____.

   Combine the digits _____, _____, _____ to create the new number of _____.

   Add the numbers _____ + _____ + _____ = _____.

2. Counting by 5: 5, 10, _____, 20, 25, _____, 35, 40, _____, 50.

   Combine the digits _____, _____, _____ to create the new number of _____.

   Add the numbers _____ + _____ + _____ = _____.

---

## MANUAL MATH CORNER

### *The Corner of Mind and Math!*

There will be times when you have to quickly perform basic math manually, there may not be a calculator nearby, there may be a power outage, or your cell phone battery may need a charge and your charger is at home. To start refreshing how to do math either in your head or on paper, start with the simple brain exercise of counting up to 100, without going over 100, in your head by 2, 5, 10, 15, 20, 25.

| |
|---|
| 2, 4, 6, 8, 10, 12, 14, 16, 18, 20, 22, 24, 26, 28, 30, 32, 34, 36, 38, 40, 42, 44, 46, 48, 50, 52, 54, 56, 58, 60, 62, 64, 66, 68, 70, 72, 74, 76, 78, 80, 82, 84, 86, 88, 90, 92, 94, 96, 98, 100. |
| 5, 10, 15, 20, 25, 30, 35, 40, 45, 50, 55, 60, 65, 70, 75, 80, 85, 90, 95, 100. |
| 10, 20, 30, 40, 50, 60, 70, 80, 90, 100. |
| 15, 30, 45, 60, 75, 90. |
| 20, 40, 60, 80, 100. |
| 25, 50, 75, 100. |

## ROMAN NUMERALS

Roman numerals use specific letters to represent numbers. Table 1-2 shows the Arabic number and the corresponding Roman numerals. By the end of this chapter, you should feel very comfortable reading and writing Roman numerals as well as converting them to Arabic numbers and Arabic numbers to Roman numerals.

**TABLE 1-2  Arabic Numbers and Roman Numerals**

| Arabic Numbers | Roman Numerals |
|:---:|:---:|
| 1/2 | ss |
| 1 | I |
| 5 | V |
| 10 | X |
| 50 | L |
| 100 | C |
| 500 | D |
| 1000 | M |

## Rules for Roman Numerals

Adding and subtracting Roman numeral letter symbols in various ways represent other numbers. There are several rules that govern the use of Roman numerals. Understanding and remembering these rules will assist allied health professionals and nurses in correctly interpreting the Roman numerals often used in lab and medication orders. In this section, we will review the following rules for Roman numerals:

1. A letter can only be repeated **THREE** times.
2. If a letter is placed **BEFORE** another letter of **greater** value, then **subtract** the smaller amount.

   Rule 2a: Only subtract powers of ten.

   Rule 2b: Only subtract **one** number from another.
3. If a letter is placed **AFTER** another letter of **greater** value, then **add** the smaller amount.

### Rule 1

1. A letter can only repeat itself **THREE** times.

---

**EXAMPLE**

**XXX = 30**

(X = 10) plus (X = 10) plus (X = 10) equals 30

X + X + X = 30

---

**EXAMPLE**

XXXX *does not* equal 40; this would be repeating a letter more than **THREE** times.

(Writing 40 will be explained later in the chapter.)

---

**Practice Exercise 1-5**  Convert the following Arabic numbers to Roman numerals.

1. 20 _____

2. 3 _____

3. 200 _____

4. 23 _____

5. 530 _____

## Rule 2

2. If a letter is placed **BEFORE** another letter of **greater** value that is **a power of 10**, then **subtract** the smaller amount.

**Another way to think about this is**: If a *smaller* number symbol is to the *left* of a larger number symbol, *subtract* the smaller number symbol.

(2a) Only subtract powers of ten (I, X, or C, **never subtract V or L**).

**Powers of ten**

I = 1
X = 10
C = 100

### EXAMPLE

IV = 4

V is *greater* than I, so *subtract* I from V

Or

I is to the *left* of V, and I is *less* than V; therefore, we *subtract*

(V = 5) *minus* (I = 1) *equals* 4

V – I = 4

### EXAMPLE

XL = 40

L is *greater* than X, so *subtract* X from L

Or

X is to the *left* of L, and X is *less* than L; therefore, we *subtract*

(L = 50) minus (X = 10) equals 40

L – X = 40

### EXAMPLE

VX *does not* equal 5

V is *not* a **power of 10**

**Practice Exercise 1-6**  Convert the following Roman numerals to Arabic numbers.

1. IX     _____
2. CM     _____
3. XCIX   _____
4. XLIV   _____
5. IV     _____

(2b) Only subtract **one** number from another.

> **EXAMPLE**
>
> **IX = 9** (10 – 1 = 9)
>
> **X is _greater_ than I, so we subtract**
>
> (X = 10) minus (I = 1) equals 9
>
> X – I = 9

> **EXAMPLE**
>
> **XC = 90** (100 – 10 = 90)
>
> **C is _greater_ than X, so we subtract**
>
> (C = 100) minus (X = 10) equals 90
>
> C – X = 90

> **EXAMPLE**
>
> IIV *does not* equal 3. **This would be subtracting <u>two</u> numbers.**
>
> **(III = 3)**

**Practice Exercise 1-7**  Convert the following Arabic numbers to Roman numerals.

1. 900  _____

2. 40  _____

3. 49  _____

4. 24  _____

5. 99  _____

## Rule 3

3. If a letter is placed **AFTER** another letter of **greater** value, then **add** the smaller amount.

**Another way to think about this is:** If a *smaller* number symbol is to the *right* of a larger number symbol, *add* the smaller number's value.

> **EXAMPLE**
>
> **VII = 7** (5 + 2 = 7)
>
> **V is _greater_ than II so we add V and II**
>
> *Or*
>
> **II is to the *right* of V, and is *less* than V; therefore, we *add***
>
> (V = 5) plus (II = 2) equals 7
>
> V + II = 7

**EXAMPLE**

**XVIII = 18** (10 + 5 + 3 = 18)

X is _greater_ than V, so add X and V

_Or_

V is to the right of X, and is _less_ than X; therefore, we _add_

V is _greater_ than III, so add V and III

_Or_

III is to the _right_ of V, and is _less_ than V; therefore, we _add_

(X = 10) plus (V = 5) plus (III = 3) equals 18

X + V + III = 18

**Practice Exercise 1-8**   Convert the following Roman numerals to Arabic numbers.

1. XXXV  _____

2. XVIII  _____

3. LV  _____

4. DXX  _____

5. LXII  _____

## Combining Roman Numerals

Combining Roman numerals is like a puzzle, to find the correct puzzle piece you need to apply the correct rule. Often one Roman numeral will use a combination of the rules, and we need to split the number up so that we can see what rules apply.

**EXAMPLE**

**LXIV = 64**

First we can split up the number into two separate parts, or pieces.

(LX = 60) and (IV = 4)

Then we can figure out which rules apply:

**L is _greater_ than X, so add L and X**

**L + X = 60**

This is RULE 3: If a letter is placed **AFTER** another letter of **greater** value, **add** the smaller amount.

**V is _greater_ than I, so subtract I from V**

**V − I = 4**

This is RULE 2: If a letter is placed **BEFORE** another letter of **greater** value that is **a power of 10**, then **subtract** the smaller amount.

RULE 2a: Only subtract powers of ten.

RULE 2b: Only subtract **one** number from another.

**I _is_ a power of 10, and we are only subtracting 1 number (I), so these rules apply as well.**

## E X A M P L E

**XCVII = 97**

First, split the number into parts or pieces.

(XC = 90) and (VII = 7)

Which rules apply?

**C is *greater* than X, so we subtract X from C**

**C − X = 90**

This is RULE 2: If a letter is placed **BEFORE** another letter of **greater** value that is **a power of 10**, then **subtract** the smaller amount.

RULE 2a: Only subtract powers of ten.

RULE 2b: **Only** subtract **one** number from another.

**X *is* a power of 10, and we are only subtracting 1 number (X), so these rules apply as well.**

**V is *greater* than II so we add V and II together**

**V + II = 7**

This is RULE 3: If a letter is placed **AFTER** another letter of **greater** value, **add** the smaller amount.

## Practice Exercise 1-9   Using the rules for Roman numerals, convert the following Roman numerals to Arabic numbers.

1. XVII _____

2. LXXX _____

3. DCCVII _____

4. XXXIX _____

5. XLII _____

## Review Exercises   Convert the following Roman numerals into Arabic numbers.

1. XL _____         6. XXXV _____

2. LXXIX _____      7. LXXXI _____

3. DI _____         8. CM _____

4. XLIV _____       9. XXXII _____

5. XCVII _____      10. LVI _____

*Convert the following Arabic numbers into Roman numerals.*

1. 80 _____         6. 51 _____

2. 890 _____        7. 44 _____

3. 7 _____          8. 20 _____

4. 76 _____         9. 38 _____

5. 24 _____         10. 1000 _____

**Now let's use our new skills for something fun!**

## Recipes for success......

### SCENARIO 1

You are planning to host the NFL Super Bowl XLVIII party at your place. Everyone is anxious to see what is on the menu this year.

You choose Chicken and Sausage Chili for the main dish. It is your Uncle Charlie's recipe and he wrote all the ingredient amounts in Roman numerals to keep it a family secret. It feeds XL, so it is perfect for this event.

*Convert the following recipe from Roman numerals to Arabic numbers.*

### Ingredients

XV (XIV and s ounces) cans of stewed tomatoes  _____

II and ss cups of beer  _____

I–II teaspoons hot sauce  _____

X beef bouillon cubes  _____

ss cup and I tablespoon brown sugar  _____

II and ss teaspoons chili powder  _____

II and ss teaspoons paprika  _____

I and ss teaspoons oregano  _____

I and ss teaspoons garlic powder  _____

ss teaspoon of cayenne pepper  _____

I tablespoon and II teaspoons of olive oil  _____

II and ss chopped red onions  _____

V lbs. ground chicken  _____

III and ss lbs. of bulk Italian sausage  _____

X (VI oz.) cans tomato paste  _____

V (XV oz.) cans kidney beans  _____

### SCENARIO 2

You are famous for your Mexican VII Layer dip, so everyone will be expecting that as well. Uncle Charlie has volunteered to make it this year if he can use your recipe. In keeping with the family tradition you e-mail it to him in Roman numerals. This recipe serves XL as well.

*Convert the following ingredients to Roman numerals.*

### Ingredients

4 lbs. of ground beef  _____

2½ (16 oz.) cans of refried beans  _____

10½ cups shredded Cheddar/Monterey Jack cheese blend  _____

2½ (8 oz.) containers of sour cream  _____

3 cups guacamole                                    _____

3 cups chunky style salsa                           _____

2½ (2 oz.) cans of chopped black olives             _____

1½ cups chopped tomato                              _____

1½ cups chopped green onion                         _____

As an Allied health professional or nurse you wouldn't be using cooking recipes, but you would see these same types of expressions in various medical settings.

### SCENARIO 3

You are a laboratory assistant and your supervisor has asked you to make a recipe card to use for making a 1 part bleach to 9 part water cleaning solution for the laboratory counter tops and blood drawing tables. You need to make ten cups of solution total. You have two gallons of distilled water and a half gallon of bleach in the lab to use to make your solution. To write the recipe for the bleach and water solution, you need to determine how much water and how much bleach will you need.

To make a 10-cup solution of 1 part bleach to 9 parts water, pour _____ cup/s water into a large spill-proof container, then slowly add _____ cup/s of bleach, secure cap tightly, mix carefully.

1. How much bleach will you need? _____

2. How much water will you need? _____

*Using the 8 steps to setting up and solving equations for story problems, solve the story problem.*

Step 1: _____

Step 2: _____

Step 3: _____

Step 4: _____

Step 5: _____

Step 6: _____

Step 7: _____

Step 8: _____

**Nursing and Numbers**

As a nurse you are involved in working with all numbering systems. Understanding numbering systems is essential in daily nurse/patient care.

Numbering is used in reading physician orders, interpretation of pharmaceutical doses to meet the need of each individual patient, to measurement of fluids and much more.

Every procedure used in the nurse/patient relationship is number related. It can start from as simple as measuring the volume of juice given to a patient to as critical as calculating intravenous drug dosing.

Be familiar with numbers and enjoy your nursing care.

## CHAPTER SUMMARY

- Numbers can be written using words, letters, digits, and symbols.
- Numbers can be written in different ways, such as whole numbers, fractions, decimals, and percentages.
- Story problems are questions that can be answered by reading a story.
- To solve story problems, information must be properly identified and extracted.
- Story problems may contain extraneous information.
- When working with story problems, it is important to be able to set up and solve mathematical equations.
- Arabic numbers are formed using the digits 0, 1, 2, 3, 4, 5, 6, 7, 8, 9.
- Arabic number digits expressed in different ways have different values.
- Roman numerals use letters to represent number values.
- Rules for Roman numerals:

  1. A letter can only be repeated **THREE** times.

  2. If a letter is placed **BEFORE** another letter of **greater** value then **subtract** the smaller amount. Note: **ONLY** subtract powers of 10.

  3. If a letter is placed **AFTER** another letter of **greater** value, then **add** the smaller amount.

## Chapter 1 Practice Test

**Read each sentence in the paragraph for numbers. Write the numbers differently using words, letters, digits, and symbols.**

The 27-year-old male patient was seen today for his 3-month postappendectomy follow-up appointment. His skin color was good, he had no complaints, his weight was 173 pounds, and his temperature was 98.4 degrees. The patient has a $25.00 co-payment for office visits.

27 years old: _____

3 months: _____

173 pounds: _____

98.4 degrees: _____

$25.00: _____

**List the 8 Steps to Setting up and Solving Equations for Story Problems:**

Step 1: _____

Step 2: _____

Step 3: _____

Step 4: _____

Step 5: _____

Step 6: _____

Step 7: _____

Step 8: _____

**Solve the Story Problems**

*Using the 8 steps to setting up and solving equations for story problems, solve the story problem.*

You are scheduled to attend a continuing education conference next weekend. The conference is out of town, and it will take you 2 hours to drive to the convention center from your home. You are expected to attend a dinner reception at 6:00 PM on Friday night at the convention center. You want to arrive early to check into your room and freshen up before the dinner reception, so you plan to arrive at 4:30 PM.

What time would you need to leave your home next Friday in order to arrive at the convention center at 4:30 PM?

Step 1: _____

Step 2: _____

Step 3: _____

Step 4: _____

Step 5: _____

Step 6: _____

Step 7: _____

Step 8: _____

**List the number of digits in each number:**

1. 47  _____
2. 253  _____
3. 019  _____
4. 15100  _____
5. 6141  _____
6. 750  _____

**Fill in the missing numbers in the counting lines:**

1. 2s: 2, 4, 6, _____, 10, 12, 14, _____, 18, 20, _____, 24, 26, 30.
2. Combine the digits _____, _____, _____ to create the new number of _____.
3. Add the numbers _____ + _____ + _____ = _____
4. 5's: 5, _____, 15, 20, _____, 30, 35, _____, 45, 50.
5. Combine the digits _____, _____, _____ to create the new number of _____.
6. Add the numbers _____ + _____ + _____ = _____
7. Express the Arabic digits 3 and 5 as a fraction.  _____
8. Express the Arabic digits 1 and 4 as a decimal.  _____

**Answer *True* or *False* to the following statements:**

1. 45 expressed as a Roman numeral is XLV  _____
2. LL (as a Roman numeral) is the correct way to express 100  _____
3. ½ is expressed ss as a Roman numeral  _____
4. If a letter is placed *BEFORE* another letter of greater value, then **add** the smaller amount  _____
5. CM equals 900  _____

**6.** 45 is a fraction    _____

**7.** A letter used as a Roman numeral can only repeat itself **THREE** times    _____

**8.** VVVVV = 25    _____

**Convert the following Arabic numbers to Roman numerals.**

**1.** 33  _____        **6.** 701  _____

**2.** 82  _____        **7.** 54  _____

**3.** 5  _____         **8.** 66  _____

**4.** 19  _____        **9.** 73  _____

**5.** 101  _____       **10.** 90  _____

**Convert the following Roman numerals to Arabic numbers.**

**1.** XLIX  _____      **6.** DL  _____

**2.** DXXX  _____      **7.** LI  _____

**3.** XV  _____        **8.** III  _____

**4.** L  _____         **9.** XVI  _____

**5.** XCIII  _____      **10.** MD  _____

# 2 Basic Operations and Whole Numbers

## INTRODUCTION

As an allied health professional or nurse, the basic math skills of adding, subtracting, multiplying and dividing are imperative skills that you will use every day. The ability to perform these basic math functions can make a difference in the overall success of the practice, as well as the life of a patient. In chapter 2, you will learn simply ways to solve basic math equations correctly and quickly. You will also learn shortcuts, as well as tips, for successfully solving multiple types of equations, and how to check your work.

## KEY TERMS

1. **Addition** A mathematical operation that represents the total or sum of two or more objects or numbers. Addition is represented in a math equation with a "plus sign" (+).

2. **Decrease** The act of taking one or more numbers or objects away from a larger amount of numbers or objects.

3. **Difference** A mathematical term to describe the answer to a subtraction equation.

4. **Division** A mathematical operation that separates the entire value of a number into multiple smaller-value parts. Division is represented in a math equation with a "division sign" (÷) or (/).

5. **Equation** A mathematical expression that contains two or more numbers, a mathematical calculation or action and a conclusion or answer.

6. **Increase** The act of adding one or more numbers to a given number.

7. **Subtraction** A mathematical operation that represents the removal or taking away of an object or number from a larger amount. Subtraction is represented in a math equation with a "minus sign" (−).

8. **Multiplication** A mathematical operation that repeats a number's value multiple times. Multiplication is represented in a math equation with a "multiplication sign" (x).

9. **Place holder** A zero (0) that is used to assist in lining numbers up in columns in a mathematical equation.

10. **Place Value** The value of a number in multiples of ten, based on the digit's placement.

11. **Product** A mathematical term to describe the answer to a multiplication equation.

12. **Quotient** A mathematical term to describe the answer to a division equation.

13. **Sum** A mathematical term to describe the answer to an addition equation.

14. **Total** The sum of two or more numbers or objects.

## LEARNING OBJECTIVES

1. Understand number place values.
2. Perform basic addition with multiple numbers.
3. Perform basic subtraction with multiple numbers.
4. Perform basic multiplication with multiple numbers.
5. Perform basic division with multiple numbers.
6. Understand multiplication tables.
7. Ability to use math shortcuts.
8. Perform basic math skills to solve story problems.
9. Ability to check your work.

# BASICS OF ADDITION

Addition is a mathematical operation that represents the **total** of two or more numbers or objects. Addition is represented in a math equation with a "plus sign" (+). Math problems are equations. Equation is a mathematical expression that contains two or more numbers, a mathematical calculation or action, and a conclusion or answer. The answer to addition equations is referred to as the sum.

In math, addition is commonly defined as the sum of two or more numbers. Addition can also be defined as:

A part being added

Or:

The result of increasing

We perform addition in our everyday lives without even knowing we are doing it. For instance, when we add one ingredient to another, in order to make a bleach solution to clean the lab counters, we have performed addition.

---

**EXAMPLE**

9 cups water

1 cup bleach

9 + 1 = 10 cups of bleach solution,

or

$$\begin{array}{r} 9 \\ +1 \\ \hline 10 \end{array}$$

Another example,

You have 16 colleagues attending a lecture on effective communication skills, and 3 colleagues ask if they can bring a guest.

16 + 3 = 19

or

$$\begin{array}{r} 16 \\ +\ 3 \\ \hline 19 \end{array}$$

So you *added* **three** more people to your attendee list. The ***sum or total*** is 19.

---

**Practice Exercise 2-1**  Solve the following addition equations.

**1.** 20 + 8  =  _____

**2.** 8 + 6  =  _____

**3.** 4 + 4  =  _____

**4.** 13 + 2  =  _____

**5.** 0 + 7  =  _____

## Adding Whole Numbers

When adding whole numbers, it is important to know that numbers have place values. A place value is the value of a number in multiples of ten, based on the digit's placement.

**Table 2-1** explains the place values of whole numbers; you can see that as you move to the *left*, the place value increases.

**TABLE 2-1  Place Values**

| Million | Hundred Thousand | Ten Thousand | Thousand | Hundred | Ten | One |
|---|---|---|---|---|---|---|
| 1,000,000 | 100,000 | 10,000 | 1000 | 100 | 10 | 1 |

**EXAMPLE**

Let's look at the place value each number holds in the number 264.

The number 264

By using the chart above,

We can see that 2 is in the *hundred's* place (2 = 200).

We can see that 6 is in the *ten's* place (6 = 60).

From the chart above we can see that 4 is in the *one's* place (4 = 4).

**EXAMPLE**

Here we can use addition.

```
  200
  060   ←┐      (Use zeros (0) as a place holder)
 +004   ←┘
  264
```

When adding whole numbers, it is important to add numbers by putting one number on top of the other in columns. This is the easiest way to add multiple numbers correctly. At this point, it doesn't matter which number is on top and which is at the bottom, but they should line up. A **place holder** is a zero that is used to assist in lining numbers up in columns in a mathematical equation. You should always use a 0 (zero) as a place holder to assist you in lining up the numbers.

**EXAMPLE**

87 + 2 = 89

```
  87
 +02   ←      (Use zero (0) as a place holder)
  89
```

In this equation, a two-digit number is on top, so we use a 0 as a placeholder to assist us in lining up the numbers.

As an allied health professional or nurse, it is very important to line your numbers up in columns so that your place values are correct.

Not lining up numbers in the correct format will not only give you an incorrect answer, it can lead to a serious medical error. Always double check your calculations, or use a calculator to make sure you did it correctly.

Now let's add some more numbers!

**EXAMPLE**

```
  234
 +044
  278
```

We always start adding from the *right* and move to the *left*.

—*Continued next page*

*Continued—*

**STEP 1** is to add the numbers in the column farthest to the *right*.

$$234$$
$$+044$$
$$\overline{\phantom{00}8}$$

*4 + 4 = 8*

**STEP 2** is to add the next column of numbers (again moving left) and put the sum directly beneath them.

$$234$$
$$+044$$
$$\overline{278}$$

*3 + 4 = 7*

**STEP 3** is to add the next column of numbers and put the sum directly beneath them.

$$234$$
$$+044$$
$$\overline{278}$$

*2 + 0 = 2*

**Practice Exercise 2-2**  Set the addition equations up using vertical columns, and then find the sum of the numbers.

**1.** 456 + 3 + 420 =

**2.** 365 + 132 =

**3.** 602 + 313 + 74 =

**4.** 703 + 20 + 5 =

**5.** 123 + 325 =

When two or more numbers add up to more than 9 we need to use the **"Carry-Over"** method to get the correct sum.

**EXAMPLE  1**

26 + 6 =

Set up the equation in columns.

$$26$$
$$+\ 06$$

**STEP 1** 6 + 6 = 12, so we would put a 2 directly below the 6 + 6 column and **"Carry-Over"** the 1 to the next column.

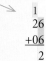
$$1$$
$$26$$
$$+06$$
$$\overline{\phantom{00}2}$$

**STEP 2** We add the **"Carried-Over"** number to the column below, so, 1 + 2 + 0 = **3**. We put that number directly below in the same column.

$$1$$
$$26$$
$$+06$$
$$\overline{32}$$

**So, *26 + 6 = 32*.**

## EXAMPLE 2

567 + 867 + 1001 =

Set up the equation in columns.

```
      567
      867
    +1001
```

**STEP 1** Here we add the far right column first of 7 + 7 + 1 = 15, so we would put a 5 directly below the 7 + 7 + 1 column and **"Carry-Over"** the 1 to the next column.

```
        1
      567
      867
    +1001
        5
```

**STEP 2** We add the **"Carried-Over"** number to the next column, so, 1 + 6 + 6 + 0 = 13. We put the 3 directly below the 6 + 6 + 1 + 0 and **"Carry-Over"** the 1 to the column to the left.

```
       11
      567
      867
    +1001
       35
```

**STEP 3** We add the **"Carried-Over"** number to the next column, 1 + 5 + 8 + 0 = 14. We put the 4 directly below the 1 + 5 + 8 + 0 and **"Carry-Over"** the 1 to the column to the left.

```
      111
      567
      867
    +1001
      435
```

**STEP 4** We add the **"Carried-Over"** number to the next column, so, 1 + 1 = 2. We add the column together and put the 2 directly below.

```
      111
      567
      867
    +1001
     2435
```

**So, 567 + 867 + 1001 = 2435**

Remember to only **Carry Over** when the numbers in the column **add up to more than 9**; otherwise just continue to the column to the *left*.

## EXAMPLE

712 + 328 =

Set up the equation in columns.

```
      712
     +328
```

—*Continued next page*

*Continued—*

**STEP 1** Here we add the far right column first, 2 + 8 = 10, so we would put a 0 directly below the 2 + 8 and **"CARRY OVER"** the 1 to the next column.

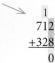

```
    1
  712
 +328
    0
```

**STEP 2** Next we add the middle column of 1 + 1 + 2 = 4. **This does not add up to more than 9 and so there is nothing to carry over.** We simply add the numbers in the column, put the 4 directly below the 1 + 1 + 2 and move *left* to the next column.

```
    1
  712
 +328
 1040
```

**STEP 3** Now we add the far left column of 7 + 3 = 10, so we would put a 10 directly below the 7 + 3. **Since there are no more numbers to the *left*, we no longer have to CARRY OVER.** We can simply add the numbers and put the sum below them.

```
    1
  712
 +328
 1040
```

## Practice Exercise 2-3   Add the following numbers using the **CARRY OVER** method; **show your work next to the equation**. Double check your answers using a calculator.

1.
```
   4531
   2551
 + 0091
```

2.
```
    002
 + 999
```

3.
```
   4871
 + 6711
```

4.
```
    194
 + 067
```

5.
```
    981
    755
 + 046
```

## SHORTCUTS

There are several shortcuts that can help you do addition "on the fly." Although these tricks assist in solving problems quickly, as an allied health professional or nurse, the best practice is to use a calculator or paper to double check your work. This will ensure that your calculations are correct.

1. **Count upward from a number**

   For example if you are adding the numbers 17 and 5, start with the larger number, **17,** and count upward 5 more to get the sum. Always start with the larger number.

   17, 18, 19, 20, 21, **22**

2. **Count by twos, fives, or tens**

   For example, if you are adding the numbers 35 and 40, start with the larger number, **40,** and count by tens and fives upward to get the sum.

   40, 50, 60, 70, **75**

   10 + 10 + 10 + 5 = 35,   40 + 35 = 75

**3. Add numbers to equal Ten**

For example, 8 and 2 equals 10. Add these together first, and count upwards 4 more to get the sum of 14.

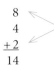

$$
\begin{array}{r}
8 \\
4 \\
+\,2 \\
\hline
14
\end{array}
$$

**4. Break up large numbers into to tens and single digit numbers.**

For example,

$$
\begin{array}{r}
13 \\
+\,02 \\
\hline
\end{array}
$$

First, break the 13 into 10 and 3.

Next add together the 3 plus 2, this equals 5.

Now add the 10.

Therefore, the sum of 13 and 2 is 15.

**Practice Exercise 2-4**   Solve the following addition equations. Line up each equation in columns. Show your work next to each problem.

1. 450 + 82 =

2. 960 + 489 =

3. 123 + 1556 =

4. 565 + 214 =

5. 43 + 678 + 89 =

6. 1433 + 9829 =

7. 56 + 811 + 9 =

8. 333 + 12 + 45 + 87 =

9. 165 + 76 + 123 + 40 =

10. 862 + 113 + 67 =

# BASICS OF SUBTRACTION

**Subtraction** is a mathematical operation that represents the removal, or taking away, of an object or number from a larger amount. Subtraction is represented in a math equation with a "minus sign" (−). The answer to subtraction equations is referred to as the difference. Difference is a mathematical term that describes the answer to a subtraction equation. Subtraction is basically the opposite of addition. It is like doing addition backwards. The best way to think about subtraction is that you are "taking something away," causing your total to decrease. To decrease a total is the act of taking one or more numbers or objects away from a larger amount of numbers or objects. For instance, the medical vehicle dealer has three ambulances for sale; your company buys two. That means he has one left. Three ambulances minus two ambulances equal one ambulance left. 3 − 2 = **1**

Just like addition, we use subtraction every day without even thinking we are doing math.

Think to yourself of an example in your daily activities where you have used subtraction.

## Subtracting Whole Numbers

When you are subtracting whole numbers, remember to always subtract the **smaller** number from a **larger** one. For example: 8 − 2 = **6**. In this problem, the eight is the **larger number** so it comes first, then we "**take away**" or remove two (the smaller number) and the remainder, or what is left, is six.

Just like addition, when you are subtracting larger numbers make sure you line up the numbers in columns. Always start with the column on the *right* and move to *left*. Subtract each column separately.

**EXAMPLE**

$75 - 23 =$

**STEP 1** Set up the equation placing the larger number on the top.

$$
\begin{array}{r}
75 \\
-\,23 \\
\end{array}
$$
⟵    (larger number on top)

**STEP 2** Subtract the bottom number from the top number in the column furthest to the *right*. Remember to subtract each column separately.

$$
\begin{array}{r}
75 \\
-\,23 \\
\hline
2 \\
\end{array}
$$
$5 - 3 = 2$

**STEP 3** Subtract the bottom number from the top number, moving left, column by column.

$$
\begin{array}{r}
75 \\
-\,23 \\
\hline
52 \\
\end{array}
$$
$7 - 2 = 5$

**Practice Exercise 2-5**  Solve the following subtraction equations.

| | | | |
|---|---|---|---|
| 1. | $\begin{array}{r} 84 \\ -\,41 \\ \hline \end{array}$ | 4. | $\begin{array}{r} 92 \\ -\,81 \\ \hline \end{array}$ |
| 2. | $\begin{array}{r} 66 \\ -\,13 \\ \hline \end{array}$ | 5. | $\begin{array}{r} 49 \\ -\,17 \\ \hline \end{array}$ |
| 3. | $\begin{array}{r} 56 \\ -\,22 \\ \hline \end{array}$ | | |

Now that we understand the easy stuff, let's move on to something a little more difficult. What if you have a problem that looks like this?

$$
\begin{array}{r}
123 \\
-\,097 \\
\hline
\end{array}
$$

In this equation, the larger number is on top, but if you try to subtract the farthest column to the right, the three is **less** than the seven. This is where we use the **"BORROWING, or REGROUPING method."** Basically you are going to take what you need from the next number.

**EXAMPLE**

**STEP 1** First, remember your **place values**. In this equation, the three is in the **one's** place, the two is in the **ten's** place, and the one is in the **hundred's** place.

123
$1 = 100$  (The 1 in the hundred's place).
$2 = 20$   (The 2 in the ten's place).
$3 = 3$    (The 3 in the one's place).

**STEP 2** Since the two has a **value** of twenty, we will **BORROW** ten from it and add it to the three.

Borrow 10 from 20 and add it 3

$$
\begin{array}{r}
1 \\
12\!3 \\
-097 \\
\hline
\end{array}
$$

$$20 - 10 = 10$$

$$
\begin{array}{r}
1\;_1 \\
12\!3 \\
-097 \\
\hline
\end{array}
$$

$$3 + 10 = 13$$

**STEP 3** Now our first column reads: 13 − 7 =

$$
\begin{array}{r}
1\,_1 \quad 13 \\
12\!3 \\
-097 \\
\hline
6
\end{array}
$$

**STEP 4** Now let's look at the next columns; remember **we borrowed ten from the twenty,** so now our next columns would actually read as: 11 − 9 = 2

$$
\begin{array}{r}
11 \quad 1\,_1 \\
12\!3 \\
-097 \\
\hline
26
\end{array}
$$

**STEP 5** Since eleven is **greater** than nine, we don't need to borrow anything; we simply do the subtraction.

$$
\begin{array}{r}
11 \\
-09 \\
\hline
2
\end{array}
$$

So we solved our equation!

$$
\begin{array}{r}
123 \\
-097 \\
\hline
26
\end{array}
$$

## Checking Your Work

Borrowing can be challenging, but there is a simple way to check that your subtraction answer is correct.

Let's use our subtraction equation from the example above.

$$
\begin{array}{r}
123 \\
-097 \\
\hline
26
\end{array}
$$

To check your answer, simply take your subtraction equation answer (26), and add it to the bottom (lesser) number in the equation (97). If you did your subtraction correctly, the answer should be your top (greater) number.

Let's check our work: 26 + 97 =

$$
\begin{array}{r}
1 \\
97 \\
+26 \\
\hline
123
\end{array}
$$

**Let's try one more to make sure we master this.**

### EXAMPLE

$764 - 137 =$

Set up the equation

$$\begin{array}{r} 764 \\ -137 \\ \hline \end{array}$$

**STEP 1**  First, remember your **place values**. In this equation the four is in the **one's** place, the six is in the **ten's** place, and the seven is in the **hundred's** place.

764
7 = 700   (The 7 in the hundred's place).
3 = 30     (The 3 in the ten's place).
4 = 4       (The 4 in the one's place).

**STEP 2**  Since the six has a **value** of sixty, we will **BORROW** ten from it and add it to the four.

Borrow 10 from 60 and add it to 4

$$\begin{array}{r} {}^{5}\phantom{0} \\ 7\cancel{6}4 \\ -137 \\ \hline \end{array}$$

*60 − 10 = 50*

$$\begin{array}{r} {}^{5}{}_{1} \\ 7\cancel{6}4 \\ -137 \\ \hline \end{array}$$

*4 + 10 = 14*

**STEP 3**  Now our first column reads: 14 − 7 =

$$\begin{array}{r} {}^{5}{}_{1}\;\;\diagup\; 14 \\ 7\cancel{6}4 \\ -137 \\ \hline 7 \end{array}$$

**STEP 4**  Now let's look at the next columns; remember **we borrowed ten from the sixty**, so now our next columns would actually read as: 5 − 3 = 2

$$\begin{array}{r} 5 \diagdown\; {}^{5}{}_{1} \\ 7\cancel{6}4 \\ -137 \\ \hline 27 \end{array}$$

**STEP 5**  Since five is **greater** than three, we don't need to borrow anything; we simply do the subtraction.

$$\begin{array}{r} 5 \\ -3 \\ \hline 2 \end{array}$$

For our last column, one is **less** than seven, so we can do simple subtraction.

$$\begin{array}{r} {}^{5}{}_{1} \\ 7\cancel{6}4 \\ -137 \\ \hline 627 \end{array}$$

We solved our equation! 764 − 137 = 627.

Let's check our work: 627 + 137 = 76**4**

$$
\begin{array}{r}
1\phantom{00} \\
627 \\
+137 \\
\hline
764
\end{array}
$$

## TIPS FOR SUCCESS

**Success Tip**  Remember your **place values**.

**Success Tip**  When borrowing, write the new number **above** to help you remember.

**Success Tip**  The **greater** (larger) number always goes on top.

**Practice Exercise 2-6**  Solve the following subtraction equations; check your work by using addition.

1.
$$
\begin{array}{r}
547 \\
-269 \\
\hline
\end{array}
$$

4.
$$
\begin{array}{r}
1857 \\
-949 \\
\hline
\end{array}
$$

2.
$$
\begin{array}{r}
898 \\
-499 \\
\hline
\end{array}
$$

5.
$$
\begin{array}{r}
375 \\
-368 \\
\hline
\end{array}
$$

3.
$$
\begin{array}{r}
765 \\
-88 \\
\hline
\end{array}
$$

Remember to double check your equations and, when possible, **use a calculator when doing math in a medical setting**.

**Practice Exercise 2-7**  Solve the following subtraction equations. Line up each equation in columns. Show your work next to each problem.

1. 67 − 56 =

2. 961 − 288 =

3. 657 − 259 =

4. 69 − 23 =

5. 4152 − 653 =

6. 148 − 52 =

7. 784 − 365 =

8. 6212 − 1989 =

9. 3571 − 755 =

10. 5840 − 2237 =

# BASICS OF MULTIPLICATION

Multiplication is a mathematical operation that repeats a number value multiple times. Multiplication is represented in a math equation with a multiplication sign (×). When solving multiplication equations, the answer is called the product. Product is a mathematical term to describe the answer to a multiplication equation.

To multiply with ease, just remember all we are doing is repeating values of numbers multiple times. This can be as basic as repeating the value of 1 three times. With multiplication, we also use addition. The two basic mathematical functions work together as a pair, especially when we multiply several digits together. To **increase** is the act of adding one or more numbers to a given number. Therefore, another way of looking at multiplication is basically counting by numbers, which increases the value of the sum each time you count, say for instance counting by twos or by fives.

**EXAMPLE**

Repeat the value of 1 three times.

Using multiplication the equation is written as: $1 \times 3 = 3$.

Using addition the equation written as: $1 + 1 + 1 = 3$.

And, counting by ones, three times is 1, 2, 3.

## Multiplication Tables

Multiplication tables are a great tool to use for basic multiplication for the numbers 1 through 9. The more we use them the easier it is for us to recall quickly which numbers multiplied by each other equal the new value. **Table 2-2** is a basic multiplication table for the numbers 1 through 9. When reading a multiplication table, you select a number in the rows and a number in the columns and follow them until they intersect. In Table 2-2, the numbers are highlighted to solve the following multiplication problem: Multiply three times six. The answer (product) is circled in red, and is 18. So using the multiplication table, we know that $3 \times 6 = 18$. This table should be studied and memorized.

**TABLE 2-2  Multiplication Table**

| × | 1 | 2 | 3 | 4 | 5 | 6 | 7 | 8 | 9 |
|---|---|---|---|---|---|---|---|---|---|
| 1 | 1 | 2 | 3 | 4 | 5 | 6 | 7 | 8 | 9 |
| 2 | 2 | 4 | 6 | 8 | 10 | 12 | 14 | 16 | 18 |
| 3 | 3 | 6 | 9 | 12 | 15 | (18) | 21 | 24 | 27 |
| 4 | 4 | 8 | 12 | 16 | 20 | 24 | 28 | 32 | 36 |
| 5 | 5 | 10 | 15 | 20 | 25 | 30 | 35 | 40 | 45 |
| 6 | 6 | 12 | 18 | 24 | 30 | 36 | 42 | 48 | 54 |
| 7 | 7 | 14 | 21 | 28 | 35 | 42 | 49 | 56 | 63 |
| 8 | 8 | 16 | 24 | 32 | 40 | 48 | 56 | 64 | 72 |
| 9 | 9 | 18 | 27 | 36 | 45 | 54 | 63 | 72 | 81 |

**Practice Exercise 2-8**   Using Table 2-2, create individual multiplication tables for the numbers 1 through 9.

| × 1 | | × 2 | | × 3 | |
|---|---|---|---|---|---|
| 1 | | 1 | | 1 | |
| 2 | | 2 | | 2 | |
| 3 | | 3 | | 3 | |
| 4 | | 4 | | 4 | |
| 5 | | 5 | | 5 | |
| 6 | | 6 | | 6 | |
| 7 | | 7 | | 7 | |
| 8 | | 8 | | 8 | |
| 9 | | 9 | | 9 | |

| ×4 | | ×5 | | ×6 | |
|---|---|---|---|---|---|
| 1 | | 1 | | 1 | |
| 2 | | 2 | | 2 | |
| 3 | | 3 | | 3 | |
| 4 | | 4 | | 4 | |
| 5 | | 5 | | 5 | |
| 6 | | 6 | | 6 | |
| 7 | | 7 | | 7 | |
| 8 | | 8 | | 8 | |
| 9 | | 9 | | 9 | |

| ×7 | | ×8 | | ×9 | |
|---|---|---|---|---|---|
| 1 | | 1 | | 1 | |
| 2 | | 2 | | 2 | |
| 3 | | 3 | | 3 | |
| 4 | | 4 | | 4 | |
| 5 | | 5 | | 5 | |
| 6 | | 6 | | 6 | |
| 7 | | 7 | | 7 | |
| 8 | | 8 | | 8 | |
| 9 | | 9 | | 9 | |

## Multiplying Whole Numbers

When multiplying whole numbers, we need to remember that all we are doing is repeating the values of numbers multiple times, and that multiplication and addition work together. Working with the numbers of 1 through 9, we will review basic multiplication using 1, 2, and 3 digits. But first let's practice various ways to repeat the value of numbers, as previously discussed in basics of multiplication.

**EXAMPLE**

What is three times six?

This is nothing more than saying that we are repeating the value of 6 three times.

When using multiplication, this is written as $3 \times 6 = 18$.

When using addition, this is written as $6 + 6 + 6 = 18$.

Counting by six three times is: 6, 12, 18.

$3 \times 6 = 18$.

Is the same as

$6 + 6 + 6 = 18$.

This is the same as counting by 6 three times: 6, 12, 18.

**Practice Exercise 2-9** Repeat the value of the numbers 1 through 9 by writing equations using multiplication and addition, and then count by the value of the number repeated by the stated number of times.

**1.** Repeat the value of 1 four times.

Multiplication:

Addition:

Counting:

**2.** Repeat the value of 2 three times.

Multiplication:

Addition:

Counting:

**3.** Repeat the value of 3 five times.

Multiplication:

Addition:

Counting:

**4.** Repeat the value of 4 two times.

Multiplication:

Addition:

Counting:

**5.** Repeat the value of 5 seven times.

Multiplication:

Addition:

Counting:

**6.** Repeat the value of 6 six times.

Multiplication:

Addition:

Counting:

**7.** Repeat the value of 7 three times.

Multiplication:

Addition:

Counting:

**8.** Repeat the value of 8 five times.

Multiplication:

Addition:

Counting:

**9.** Repeat the value of 9 four times.

Multiplication:

Addition:

Counting:

Remember, multiplication problems can be solved in different ways. Working with the format that works best for you is the key to successfully solving multiplication equations. We will look at two different ways to solve multiplication equations. Once you determine which format works best for you, stick with it! When you are multiplying large numbers or numbers larger than 9, you need to multiply each number separately. Just like addition, the numbers need to line up correctly in columns. Then just add the answers from each column together.

Let's set up equations for three multiplication problems using 1, 2, and 3 digits to express ones, tens, and hundreds place values.

## TIPS FOR SUCCESS

**Success Tip** Remember the place value chart from the **addition section** of this chapter.

| Million | Hundred Thousand | Ten Thousand | Thousand | Hundred | Ten | One |
|---------|------------------|--------------|----------|---------|-----|-----|
| 1,000,000 | 100,000 | 10,000 | 1000 | 100 | 10 | 1 |

**Success Tip** Remember to use 0 as a place holder when adding multiple numbers, so that the place value columns line up (go back to the **addition section** of this chapter if you need a refresher).

## EXAMPLE

Let's look at the place value each number holds in the number 453.

**1.** Multiply 1 by 3 (The 3 is the one place value).

**2.** Multiply 10 by 5 (The 5 is the ten place value).

**3.** Multiply 100 by 4 (The 4 is the hundred place value).

**EXAMPLE  1**

Multiply 1 by 3.    $1 \times 3 = 3$

$$
\begin{array}{r}
1 \\
\underline{\times 3} \\
3
\end{array}
$$

**EXAMPLE  2**

Multiply 10 by 5.    $10 \times 5 = 50$

$$
\begin{array}{r}
10 \\
\underline{\times 05} \\
50
\end{array}
$$   ⟵    (use zeros as place holders so the place value columns line up)

**EXAMPLE  3**

Multiply 100 by 4.    $100 \times 4 = 400$

$$
\begin{array}{r}
100 \\
\underline{\times 004} \\
400
\end{array}
$$   ⟵    (use zeros as place holders so the place value columns line up)

Now, let's put them together:

Working from highest value to lowest value this is done by adding:

$400 + 50 = 450$, and $450 + 3 = 453$

$$
\begin{array}{r}
400 \\
050 \\
\underline{+\,003} \\
453
\end{array}
$$   ⟵    (use zeros as place holders so the place value columns line up)

Working from lowest value to highest value is:

$3 + 50 = 53$, and $53 + 400 = 453$

$$
\begin{array}{r}
003 \\
050 \\
\underline{+\,400} \\
453
\end{array}
$$   ⟵    (use zeros as place holders so the place value columns line up)

Now let's try multiplying three hundred and twenty one by two.

**EXAMPLE**

Multiply 321 by 2.

**STEP 1**  Set up your equation

$$
\begin{array}{r}
321 \\
\underline{\times 002}
\end{array}
$$   ⟵    (use zeros as place holders so the place value columns line up)

**STEP 2**  Here we start with the ones place (lowest value).

$1 \times 2 = 2$

$$
\begin{array}{r}
321 \\
\underline{\times 002} \\
2
\end{array}
$$   ⟵    (use zeros as place holders so the place value columns line up)

*—Continued next page*

*Continued—*

**STEP 3** Then, the tens place $20 \times 2 = 40$

```
    321
  ×002  ←┐
    002  ←┘      (use zeros as place holders so the place value columns line up)
    040
```

**STEP 4** And last, the hundreds place (highest value). $300 \times 2 = 600$

```
    353
  ×002  ←┐
    002  ←┘      (use zeros as place holders so the place value columns line up)
    040
    600
```

**STEP 5** Now all we have to do is **add** the three answers together:

Working from highest value to lowest value this is done by adding:

$600 + 40 = 640$, and $640 + 2 = 642$  or,

```
    600
    040  ←┐
  +002  ←┘      (use zeros as place holders so the place value columns line up)
    642
```

Working from lowest value to highest value is:

$2 + 40 = 42$, and $42 + 600 = 642$ or,

```
    002  ←┐
    040  ←┘      (use zeros as place holders so the place value columns line up)
  +600
    642
```

Now let's try one where we have to carry a number over to the next value place. When multiplying, like with addition, there are times when our product of a place value is greater than the number value. When two or more numbers add up to more than 9, we need to use the "Carry-Over" method to get the correct product.

---

**EXAMPLE**

Multiply 453 by 4.

**STEP 1** Set up the equation.

```
    453
  ×004
```

**STEP 2** Start with the one's place, $4 \times 3 = 12$, and carry the 1 over to the tens place.

```
   21
    453
  ×004
    002
```

**STEP 3** Next the ten's place, $4 \times 5 = 20 + 1 = 21$, and carry the 2 over to the hundreds place.

```
   21
    453
  ×004
    002
    010
```

**STEP 4** Now the hundred's place, $4 \times 4 = 16 + 2 = 18$.

$$
\begin{array}{r}
2\,1 \\
453 \\
\times\,004 \\
\hline
002 \\
010 \\
+1800 \\
\end{array}
$$

**STEP 5** Now, we add to solve our equation.

$$
\begin{array}{r}
2\,1 \\
453 \\
\times\,004 \\
\hline
002 \\
010 \\
+1800 \\
\hline
1812 \\
\end{array}
$$

Or, you can work each separately and then simply add:

$453 \times 4 =$

$4 \times 3 = 12$

$4 \times 50 = 200$

$4 \times 400 = 1600$

Now, add to find your product

$1600 + 200 = 1800,$ *and* $1800 + 12 = 1812$

Or,

$$
\begin{array}{r}
1600 \\
0200 \\
+0012 \\
\hline
1812 \\
\end{array}
$$

**Practice Exercise 2-10** Solve the following multiplication problems.

1. $2 \times 5 =$

2. $7 \times 9 =$

3. $10 \times 4 =$

4. $15 \times 5 =$

5. $12 \times 7 =$

6. $25 \times 10 =$

7. $100 \times 50 =$

8. $47 \times 20 =$

9. $250 \times 3 =$

10. $60 \times 3 =$

## SHORTCUTS

Now that you have refreshed your memory on how to multiply, remember the shortcuts we covered. These shortcuts are counting by the value of a number, working each value place separately, and then simply adding them together.

A few fun facts about the multiples of 9 is that as you count by the value of 9, each value increases in the tens place by one and decreases in the ones place by one, and when you add the digits of the ones and tens place together they always equal 9.

| Multiples of 9 | 09 | 18 | 27 | 36 | 45 | 54 | 63 | 72 | 81 | 90 |
|---|---|---|---|---|---|---|---|---|---|---|
| **Tens** | 0 | 1 | 2 | 3 | 4 | 5 | 6 | 7 | 8 | 9 |
| **Ones** | 9 | 8 | 7 | 6 | 5 | 4 | 3 | 2 | 1 | 0 |
| **Digits** | 0+9=9 | 1+8=9 | 2+7=9 | 3+6=9 | 4+5=9 | 5+4=9 | 6+3=9 | 7+2=9 | 8+1=9 | 9+0=9 |

# BASICS OF DIVISION

Division is a mathematical operation that separates the entire value of a number into multiple smaller-value parts. Division is represented in a math equation with a (÷) or (/). Division is the opposite of multiplication and basically simply involves separating the entire value of a number into multiple smaller number value parts, An example is cutting 1 pie into 8 pieces. When working with division problems, the answer is called the quotient. The quotient is the mathematical term to describe the answer to a division equation.

## Dividing Whole Numbers

When working with whole numbers, division is nothing more than breaking a number into groups of smaller numbers. Basically, you are simply trying to find out how many multiples of one number is in another number. Like subtraction being the opposite of addition, division is the opposite of multiplication. If you have mastered your times tables, it will help you work division with ease. Let's say that that a pharmaceutical company brings 20 ink pens to your office and you have 10 employees. You want to divide the pens up equally between the employees. How many ink pens will each employee get?

### EXAMPLE

Divide 20 ink pens by 10 employees.

$20 \div 10 = 2$. When dividing 20 by 10 we are basically taking 20 items and separating them into groups of 10.

You can also perform division using the subtraction method. This can be done by subtracting the number you are dividing by from the number you are dividing, multiple times, until you can't subtract by the number you are dividing by anymore.

### EXAMPLE

$20 \div 10 =$

$20 - 10 = 10, 10 - 10 = 0$

$\qquad\quad \uparrow \qquad\qquad\quad \uparrow$

$\qquad\quad 1 \qquad\qquad\quad 2$

Here we subtracted 10 from 20 two times to get to zero. $20 \div 10 = 2$

When working with division, your quotient will not always come out even. When this happens we need to record our answer using a remainder, which is written with an "r" in front of the remaining value.

### EXAMPLE

$25 \div 10 = 2\ \mathbf{r}\ 5$

Let's work this using the subtraction method.

$25 - 10 = 15,\ and\ 15 - 10 = 5$

$\qquad\quad \uparrow \qquad\qquad\qquad\quad \uparrow$

$\qquad\quad 1 \qquad\qquad\qquad\quad 2 \qquad\qquad$ Remainder of 5

Here we were able to subtract 10 from 25 two times, and had a remainder of 5.

## Checking Your Work

When working with division you can easily check your work by using multiplication.

Using our ink pen example above, we know that 20 ÷ 10 = 2.

To check your work, you can multiply your quotient of 2 by the number you divided by 10:

    20 ÷ 10 = 2 *is equal to* 2 × 10 = 20.

Checking your work, quotients with remainders.

Let's review our example 25 ÷ 10 = 2 **r** 5, using the subtraction method, and check our work using multiplication and addition.

---

**E X A M P L E**

25 ÷ 10 = 2 **r** 5

25 − 10 = 15, *and* 15 − 10 = 5

     ↑           ↑

     1           2       Remainder of 5

Here we were able to subtract 10 from 25 two times, and had a remainder of 5.

So, *we can multiply* 10 × 2, *which equals* 20, *and then add our remainder of* 5.

Let's check our work:

10 × 2 = 20, *and* 20 + r 5 = 25.

Our work checks out, our quotient of 2 **r** 5 for the division problem 25 ÷ 10 is correct.

---

**Practice Exercise 2-11**   Solve the following division equations; also write the multiplication and addition equations used to check your work.

  **1.** 75 ÷ 15 =

  **2.** 842 ÷ 4 =

  **3.** 37 ÷ 3 =

  **4.** 250 ÷ 50 =

  **5.** 56 ÷ 8 =

  **6.** 749 ÷ 100 =

  **7.** 144 ÷ 12 =

  **8.** 480 ÷ 30 =

  **9.** 81 ÷ 9 =

**10.** 17 ÷ 4 =

### The Corner of Mind and Math!

Using all of the tips for success and shortcuts we learned in this chapter, solve the following equations and time yourself. See if you can answer all of them in your head, correctly, in less than 60 seconds. Then rework them on paper and don't forget to check your work.

1. $8 + 4 + 2 =$
2. $13 + 2 =$
3. $75 - 40 =$

4. $453 \times 2 =$
5. $15 \times 5 =$
6. $73 \div 9 =$

**Now let's use our new skills for something fun!**

## Recipes for success......

### SCENARIO 1

Your medical office just moved to a bigger facility and is having a potluck to celebrate the move. All patients and their families are invited. That means you will need to really step up the quantities of your recipes. You volunteer to prepare Berry-bars.

### Berry-bars (serves 15)

This recipe serves 15 so you will need to multiply the quantities to feed approximately 45 people. How many times do you have to multiply your original recipe by to make enough Berry-bars? Let's divide our number of people by the servings per recipe to find out. $45 \div 15 = 3$.

*Multiply* the following ingredients to serve 45.

### Ingredients

3 cups flour                    _____

1½ cup sugar                    _____

1 egg                           _____

1 cup vegetable shortening _____

1 teaspoon salt                 _____

1 pinch of cinnamon             _____

3 teaspoons cornstarch          _____

1 teaspoon baking powder _____

4 cups of blackberries          _____

As an allied health professional or nurse you will not be using cooking recipes, but you will see these same types of equations in various medical settings.

### SCENARIO 2

Your office manager's birthday is today and the staff ordered lunch to celebrate the occasion. The bill for the office manager's birthday luncheon came to $48.00. There are 4 employees sharing the cost of the bill evenly.

How much does each employee owe for the bill? _____

**Nursing and Numbers**

As a nurse, the use of addition, subtraction, multiplication, and division are an essential part of quality patient care.

Number placement is a building block for all mathematical equations.

Learning the basics of addition, subtraction, multiplication, and division early in this process will guarantee you an easier tomorrow. These skills are the cornerstone of mathematics.

The multiplication table is essential. As a nurse, one cannot emphasize enough the need to memorize this table.

Memorizing multiplication tables will make math easier and a much more enjoyable task.

## CHAPTER SUMMARY

- All numbers have place values.
- Place value increases as you move to the *left*.
- Line up whole numbers in columns to assist in solving equations.
- Use zeros for place holders.
- Always solve the columned equation by starting with the far *right* column and move to the *left*.
- Always subtract a smaller number from a larger number.
- Subtraction is the opposite of addition.
- Use addition to double check your subtraction equation.
- Multiplication is the repeating of number values multiple times.
- Multiplication tables are a tool to solve basic equations for the numbers 1 through 9.
- Multiplication and addition work together.
- Division is the opposite of multiplication.
- Division is breaking a number into groups of smaller numbers.
- Use multiplication to double check your quotient.
- Quotients do not always come out even, leaving a "remainder."

## Chapter 2 Practice Test

Answer *True* or *False* to the following statements:

1. Lining up your numbers in columns is not important in adding or subtracting whole numbers.    _____

2. The "Product" of an equation refers to the answer of a division math problem.    _____

3. Multiplying whole numbers is the act of repeating the values of numbers multiple times.    _____

4. Multiplication and addition work together.    _____

5. Zero can be used as a place holder.    _____

6. "Borrowing" or "Regrouping" is a term used in multiplying whole numbers.    _____

7. Numbers have place values.    _____

8. We always move from left to right when solving equations.    _____

9. The larger number always goes at the bottom in a subtraction equation.    _____

10. Use multiplication to double check a quotient.    _____

**Solve the following equations. Line them up in columns and show your work next to them.**
Double check your answers using a calculator.

1. $88 + 65 =$
2. $943 - 637 =$
3. $29 \times 47 =$
4. $7 \times 20 =$
5. $233 \div 6 =$
6. $790 \times 16 =$
7. $253 - 53 =$
8. $533 - 186 =$
9. $169 + 443 =$
10. $562 \times 13 =$

11. $2345 + 123 =$
12. $84 \times 21 =$
13. $569 - 279 =$
14. $652 - 231 =$
15. $712 + 745 =$
16. $200 \times 76 =$
17. $214 + 89 =$
18. $1111 \times 85 =$
19. $432 - 254 =$
20. $96 \times 417 =$

**Solve the following equations. Use multiplication to check your answer.**
Show your work next to each problem.

1. $843 \div 82 =$
2. $984 \div 60 =$
3. $854 \div 2 =$
4. $199 \div 10 =$

5. $655 \div 5 =$
6. $754 \div 65 =$
7. $240 \div 12 =$
8. $989 \div 7 =$

**Using your skills from chapter one, solve the following equations.**
**WRITE YOUR ANSWERS IN ROMAN NUMERALS.**

1. XXIV + LVI =
2. CM − XLV =
3. XL × XIX =

**Solve the Story Problem**

You are asked to conduct inventory on the medical supply room. Your supervisor gives you a list of the minimum number of each item that needs to be on hand at all times. You are to inform her if any items fall below the minimum number and by how many. You inventory the gloves first. The minimum number of boxes of small gloves is 6, medium gloves is 8, and large gloves is 10. In the supply room, you count 6 boxes of large gloves, 5 boxes of small gloves and 9 boxes of medium gloves.

1. Do the number of boxes of large gloves fall below the minimum number required to have on hand? _____ If so, by how many boxes? _____

2. Do the number of boxes of medium gloves fall below the minimum number required to have on hand? _____ If so, by how many boxes? _____

3. Do the number of boxes of small gloves fall below the minimum number required to have on hand? _____ If so, by how many boxes? _____
What is the total number of boxes of gloves below the minimum number required? _____

# 3 Fractions and Mixed Numbers

## INTRODUCTION

A fraction is basically a whole number split into equal parts. The easiest way to picture a fraction in your mind is to think of a pie. If you cut the pie into eight pieces, each piece is one part, which is a fraction, of the whole amount. If we eat one piece of pie, we have eaten one-eighth, or $\frac{1}{8}$ of the pie. As an allied health professional or nurse, it is important to understand and do calculations with different types of fractions. **Remember to do medical math problems with a calculator whenever possible to avoid making an error.**

### KEY TERMS

1. **Denominator** A mathematical term used to identify and describe the bottom number of a fraction. The *total of all parts*, as represented in a fraction.
2. **Fraction** Any number of parts of a whole number or object.
3. **Improper Fraction** A mathematical term used to identify and describe a fraction that has a larger number as the numerator (top number) and a smaller number as the denominator (bottom number).
4. **Lowest Terms** The action of reducing (dividing) a larger fraction to its lowest possible term or represented value.
5. **Mixed Numbers** A mathematical expression using a whole number and a fraction, often converted from an improper fraction.
6. **Numerator** A mathematical term used to identify and describe the top number of a fraction. The amount of parts you *have*, as represented in a fraction.
7. **Proper Fraction** A mathematical term used to identify and describe a fraction that has a smaller number as the numerator (top number) and a larger number as the denominator (bottom number). Often reduced to lowest terms.

## FRACTIONS

A fraction is any number of parts of a whole number or object. Fractions have two values, a numerator and a denominator, which are separated by a fraction bar.

$$\frac{Numerator}{Denominator}$$

The numerator is always the value listed on top of the fraction bar and the denominator is always the value on the bottom of the fraction bar. The numerator represents a part or portion of the whole, and the denominator represents the total amount in the whole.

Fractions are usually expressed in the following ways:

$$\frac{numerator}{denominator} \quad \text{Or} \quad numerator/_{denominator}$$

There are three basic types of fractions:

**Proper Fractions**

**Improper Fractions**

**Mixed Numbers**

By the end of this chapter you will be very comfortable with all three of these and how they function.

## Proper Fractions

The box below has eight sections or parts. In a fraction, 8 would be the *denominator* or bottom number because it is the total of <u>all the parts together</u> or the whole box.

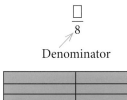

Denominator

We take one of the sections or parts away. Now the number of sections we *have* are seven sections of the **total** eight sections. The seven would be the *numerator* or top number in a fraction.

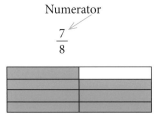

The fraction $\frac{7}{8}$ is known as a *proper fraction*. A proper fraction always has a **smaller** number as the numerator, or top number, and a **larger** number as the denominator or bottom number.

Let's look at one more to make sure we understand.

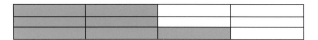

The entire block has twelve sections, so we have twelve sections **total**. Therefore, our denominator would be 12.

Seven of our sections are blue, so that is the amount or parts we *have*, making 7 the numerator.

So our proper fraction would look like this: $\frac{7}{12}$.

$$\frac{7 \; numerator}{12 \; denominator}$$

**Practice Exercise 3-1** Express the following as a proper fraction. Use the blue highlighted sections as the numerator and the total as the denominator.

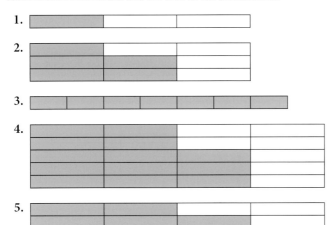

## Improper Fractions

Now that we understand a proper fraction, it is easy to guess what is meant by an *improper fraction*. An improper fraction is expressed with a **larger or equal number** as the numerator and a **smaller or equal number** as the denominator. So an improper fraction would look like this:

$$\frac{9 \; numerator}{8 \; denominator} \quad \text{Or} \quad \frac{8 \; numerator}{8 \; denominator}$$

It is fine to express your fraction this way. In fact, it is often useful when we are adding, subtracting, multiplying, or dividing fractions. We will discuss those functions in depth in the next chapter, but for now, the need is to understand the definition of an improper fraction. Let's use two square pizzas to explain an improper fraction.

Each of the two pizzas is cut into 4 pieces. Therefore, each piece is one-fourth, or $\frac{1}{4}$ of each whole pizza. Between the two pizzas, we have a total of 8 fourths, or $\frac{8}{4}$. If one piece of pizza is eaten, you have seven-fourths, or $\frac{7}{4}$, remaining.

PIZZA 1

PIZZA 2

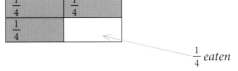

**Practice Exercise 3-2** Express the following as an improper fraction.

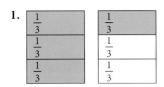

**2.**

| $\frac{1}{5}$ | $\frac{1}{5}$ | $\frac{1}{5}$ | $\frac{1}{5}$ | $\frac{1}{5}$ |

| $\frac{1}{5}$ | $\frac{1}{5}$ | $\frac{1}{5}$ | $\frac{1}{5}$ | $\frac{1}{5}$ |

**3.**

| $\frac{1}{6}$ | $\frac{1}{6}$ |   | $\frac{1}{6}$ | $\frac{1}{6}$ |
| $\frac{1}{6}$ | $\frac{1}{6}$ |   | $\frac{1}{6}$ | $\frac{1}{6}$ |
| $\frac{1}{6}$ | $\frac{1}{6}$ |   | $\frac{1}{6}$ | $\frac{1}{6}$ |

**4.**

| $\frac{1}{8}$ | $\frac{1}{8}$ | $\frac{1}{8}$ | $\frac{1}{8}$ |
| $\frac{1}{8}$ | $\frac{1}{8}$ | $\frac{1}{8}$ | $\frac{1}{8}$ |

| $\frac{1}{8}$ | $\frac{1}{8}$ | $\frac{1}{8}$ | $\frac{1}{8}$ |
| $\frac{1}{8}$ | $\frac{1}{8}$ | $\frac{1}{8}$ | $\frac{1}{8}$ |

**5.**

| $\frac{1}{2}$ | $\frac{1}{2}$ |

| $\frac{1}{2}$ | $\frac{1}{2}$ |

# MIXED NUMBERS

A **mixed number** is a mathematical expression using a whole number and a fraction, often converted from an improper fraction. Basically, a mixed number is another way to express an improper fraction. Let's use those square pizzas one more time to help us understand.

PIZZA 1

| $\frac{1}{4}$ | $\frac{1}{4}$ |
| $\frac{1}{4}$ | $\frac{1}{4}$ |

PIZZA 2

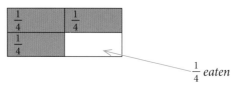

$\frac{1}{4}$ *eaten*

We take our fraction, $\frac{7}{4}$, and **divide** our numerator by our denominator.

$$7 \div 4 = 1 \text{ with a remainder of } 3$$

Take the remainder of 3, and write it as the numerator of a fraction, using your **original denominator of 4**, and write it to the right of your whole number of 1.

So your mixed number would be $1\frac{3}{4}$.

In other words, you have one and three-fourths pizza left to eat. Both expressions are correct and it is very easy to convert back to the improper fractions. This is how you can check your work. Take your denominator (4) and multiply it by the whole number (1).

$1\frac{3}{4}$

$$4 \times 1 = 4$$

Then add your remainder (3), and put the total over your **original denominator.**

$$4 + 3 = \frac{7}{4}$$

Let's do another to make sure we have mastered this.

---

### EXAMPLE

$\frac{12}{5}$

**STEP 1** Divide your numerator by the denominator.

   $12 \div 5 = 2$, *with a remainder* 2

**STEP 2** Write your whole number.

   2

**STEP 3** Write your remainder as the numerator of a fraction, using your original denominator of 5.

   $\frac{2}{5}$

So our mixed number is

   $2\frac{2}{5}$

---

Now we **multiply** to get back to our original fraction to check our work.

---

### EXAMPLE

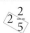 $2\frac{2}{5}$

**STEP 1** Multiply the denominator and the whole number.

   $5 \times 2 = 10$

**STEP 2** Add the remainder to the product.

   $10 + 2 = 12$

**STEP 3** Write the sum as a fraction using the original denominator.

   $\frac{12}{5}$

Great job!

---

**Practice Exercise 3-3**   Convert the following improper fractions to mixed numbers.

1. $\frac{18}{12}$            4. $\frac{10}{10}$

2. $\frac{9}{5}$             5. $\frac{23}{7}$

3. $\frac{7}{2}$

**Practice Exercise 3-4**   Convert the following mixed numbers to improper fractions.

1. $5\frac{3}{4}$

2. $3\frac{7}{12}$

3. $2\frac{6}{7}$

4. $1\frac{15}{16}$

5. $9\frac{1}{3}$

# REDUCING FRACTIONS TO LOWEST TERMS

If the numerator and the denominator of a fraction are both *evenly* divisible by the same number, other than the number one (1), the fraction can be reduced. Reducing a fraction to its lowest terms is the action of reducing (dividing) a larger fraction to its smallest represented value. In math, it is always best to reduce your fractions down to the lowest denominator. Knowing your multiplication tables will make this process much easier.

Let's take the fraction: $\frac{3}{9}$

What number are **both** three and nine evenly divisible by?

Three can be divided by three.          $3 \div 3 = 1$

Nine can be divided by three.          $9 \div 3 = 3$

Can we divide it down any further?

No. The only number that one and three can be divided by is **one**.

Our fraction becomes $\frac{1}{3}$.

That means; $\frac{3}{9} = \frac{1}{3}$

Therefore, our original fraction of $\frac{3}{9}$ reduced to the **lowest term** is $\frac{1}{3}$.

Let's try this again.

---

### EXAMPLE

In this case we will use the fraction:

$$\frac{15}{20}$$

Ask yourself what number can you divide both 15 and 20 by evenly?

How about 2?

You can divide 20 by two evenly, but not 15.

$$20 \div 2 = 10$$
$$15 \div 2 = 7\ r1$$

**To be correct we can't have a remainder.**

How about 3?

You can divide 15 by three evenly, but not 20.

$$15 \div 3 = 5$$
$$20 \div 3 = 5\ r5$$

**This is where multiplication can come in handy.** If we know our multiplication tables,

We would know that $3 \times 5 = 15$ and $4 \times 5 = 20$.

**This tells us that both 15 and 20 are evenly divisible by 5.**

Now we can reduce our fraction!

$$15 \div 5 = 3$$
$$20 \div 5 = 4$$
$$\frac{15}{20} = \frac{3}{4}$$

Sometimes we can reduce our fraction and then reduce it again. Make sure you take the fraction down as far as it will go to ensure your fraction is in lowest terms. This is called reducing the fraction to the lowest denominator or lowest terms.

### EXAMPLE

Our fraction is $\dfrac{14}{56}$.

Using our knowledge of multiplication and division, we know that 14 and 56 are both evenly divisible by 7.

$$14 \div 7 = 2$$
$$56 \div 7 = 8$$

This means our reduced fraction is $\dfrac{2}{8}$.

Can we divide that down even more?

You bet! 2 and 8 are both evenly divisible by 2. So here we go again!

$$2 \div 2 = 1$$
$$8 \div 2 = 4$$

So our lowest-term fraction is $\dfrac{1}{4}$.

**Practice Exercise 3-5**  Reduce the fractions to lowest terms.

1. $\dfrac{16}{20}$

2. $\dfrac{18}{27}$

3. $\dfrac{20}{25}$

4. $\dfrac{3}{36}$

5. $\dfrac{33}{88}$

## Recipes for success......

### SCENARIO 1

Your nutrition class is hosting an event at the local high school. To promote healthy eating, your group decides to make fruit pizza.

**Fruit Pizza (Each pizza yields eight pieces)**

1 package roll out sugar cookie dough

40 strawberries

40 blueberries

2 Kiwis sliced into 10 pieces each

24 raspberries or boysenberries

1 peach or nectarine sliced into 8 wedges

8 oz. vanilla yogurt

¼ cup honey

You are hosting two classes and each student will receive one piece of fruit pizza.

Class A has 28 students.

Class B has 30 students.

1. How many whole pizzas do you need to feed the Class A?    _____

2. How many whole pizzas do you need to feed both classes?    _____

3. Show the total students and the total pieces as a fraction for Class A.    _____

4. Reduce the fraction to lowest terms.    _____

5. Two-thirds $\left(\frac{2}{3}\right)$ of Class B ate a piece of the pizza, how many students did NOT eat a piece.    _____

6. Based on the recipe, how many strawberries are on each piece? Show your answer as fraction. Use your total strawberries as the denominator.    _____

7. Reduce your fraction to lowest terms.    _____

### SCENARIO 2

Your office is holding a chili cook-off fund raiser. It plans to donate the proceeds to the local health department for a free immunization clinic day for uninsured children. Your office manager asks that all chili recipes are healthy and that at least 7 people make chili for the event. Each person will need to make enough chili for 20 people, and each participant will be given a 4-ounce (1/2 cup) serving. You decide to make low-sodium turkey chili. Your recipe makes approximately ten 4-ounce (1/2 cup) servings. A total of 9 people have volunteered to make chili for the event. All participants are asked to make a $5.00 donation, and asked to vote for their favorite healthy chili recipe. The event is expected to have 120 to 150 participants.

1. You need to make 20 servings of chili and your recipe makes 10 servings. Write a fraction using the number of servings your chili recipe makes as the numerator and the total number of servings you have to make for the chili cook-off as the denominator, and then reduce it to lowest terms.    _____

2. How many total servings of chili will the 9 people make together? Write your answer as an improper fraction using the total number of servings as the numerator and the number of people making chili as the denominator, and then convert your answer into a proper fraction, mixed number, or whole number.    _____

3. How much money will be raised if the event has 143 participants? Write your answer as an improper fraction, and then convert your answer into a proper fraction, mixed number or whole number.    _____

### Low-Sodium Turkey Chili (makes ten ½-cup servings). How much of each ingredient is needed to make twenty ½-cup servings?

1½ pounds ground turkey (browned, rinsed, and drained well)    _____

2 15-ounce cans tomato sauce    _____

1 15-ounce can no-salt-added diced tomatoes    _____

1 16-ounce can reduced-sodium dark-red kidney beans (undrained)    _____

½ cup cold water    _____

½ teaspoon sugar    _____

½ teaspoon Hungarian paprika    _____

1 tablespoons unsweetened cocoa powder    _____

1 packet low-sodium chili spice mix    _____

**Nursing and Numbers**

A nurse will be using fractions or portions on a daily basis.

Portions can appear as "a fraction of something."

An example is an order that reads: "give ¼ of the 500 mL solution." Understanding fractions will help simplify your daily use of math.

# CHAPTER SUMMARY

- A fraction represents an equal part or parts of a whole object or number.
- The top number of a fraction is called a *numerator* and represents the amount of parts you *HAVE*.
- The bottom number of a fraction is called a *denominator*, and represents the TOTAL of all parts.
- There are three types of fractions:

  1. Proper fraction

  2. Improper fraction

  3. Mixed number

- Proper fractions have a smaller number as a numerator and a larger number as a denominator.
- Improper fractions have a larger or equal number as a numerator and a smaller or equal number as a denominator.
- Mixed numbers are another way to express an improper fraction.
- Mixed numbers use a whole number and a fraction together.
- Multiplication and division are important concepts used when working with fractions.
- The correct way to express a fraction is in the lowest form or lowest term.
- Always use a calculator to do math in a medical setting.

## Chapter 3 Practice Test

**Answer *True* or *False* to the following statements:**

1. Mixed numbers are expressed using a whole number and a fraction. _____

2. The TOTAL number of parts in a fraction is known as a numerator. _____

3. You never need to use division or multiplication when working with fractions. _____

4. A proper fraction has a larger number as the numerator and smaller number as the denominator. _____

5. The proper way to express a fraction is in the lowest terms. _____

6. To convert a fraction to lowest terms, both the numerator and the denominator have to be divisible by the same number, other than one. _____

**Express the following as a Proper Fraction. Use the highlighted sections as the numerator. If applicable reduce to the lowest terms.**

1.

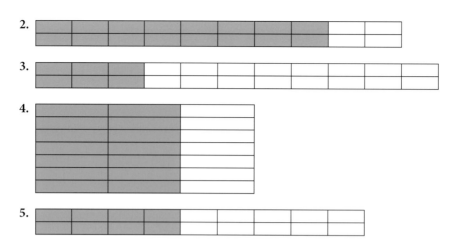

**2.**

**3.**

**4.**

**5.**

Convert the following Improper Fractions to Mixed Numbers and reduce to the lowest terms.

1. $\frac{83}{44}$ _____

2. $\frac{35}{16}$ _____

3. $\frac{67}{20}$ _____

4. $\frac{96}{25}$ _____

5. $\frac{88}{87}$ _____

6. $\frac{144}{13}$ _____

7. $\frac{75}{4}$ _____

8. $\frac{9}{5}$ _____

Convert the following Mixed Numbers to Improper Fractions.

1. $3\frac{2}{12}$ _____

2. $2\frac{2}{5}$ _____

3. $7\frac{6}{8}$ _____

4. $1\frac{12}{13}$ _____

5. $4\frac{5}{9}$ _____

6. $1\frac{2}{12}$ _____

7. $2\frac{4}{19}$ _____

8. $5\frac{2}{3}$ _____

Reduce the following fractions to the lowest terms.

1. $\frac{12}{36}$ _____

2. $\frac{42}{48}$ _____

3. $\frac{72}{144}$ _____

4. $\frac{30}{36}$ _____

5. $\frac{14}{56}$ _____

6. $\frac{3}{9}$ _____

7. $\frac{9}{27}$ _____

8. $\frac{10}{50}$ _____

**Solve the Story Problem**

Your office chili cook-off fund raiser was a success, and raised $715.00. Your office manager plans to donate the proceeds to the local health department for a free immunization clinic for uninsured children. The health department hopes to give 150 children up to 4 immunizations each. Another local business donated enough money to purchase vaccine to inoculate 40 children. The cost per immunization averages $6.50.

1. Write an improper fraction for the number of immunizations per child. _____

2. How much will it cost to give 150 children 4 immunizations each? Write your answer as an improper fraction, and then convert your answer into a proper fraction, mixed number, or whole number. _____

3. How many immunizations will your office donation provide? _____

4. Write a mixed number for the total number of children who can receive 4 immunizations each from the immunizations provided from your office donation. Remember to reduce to the lowest terms. _____

# 4 Basic Operations with Fractions

## INTRODUCTION

Now that we have an understanding of how fractions work, we need to learn how to solve basic math equations using fractions. There are specific concepts used for adding, subtracting, multiplying, and dividing fractions. It is very important to understand and remember all the concepts and when to use them. Whatever medical field you choose as a career, understanding fractions and how to complete basic operations correctly will aid in quality patient care. **Remember to always use a calculator when doing any math in a medical setting and always double-check your calculations to make sure they are correct.**

### LEARNING OBJECTIVES

1. Understand and perform addition of fractions and mixed numbers.
2. Understand and perform subtraction of fractions and mixed numbers.
3. Understand and perform multiplication of fractions and mixed numbers.
4. Understand and perform division of fractions and mixed numbers.

### KEY TERMS

1. **Common Denominator** The number quantity by which all denominators in a set of fractions may be divided evenly. Used in addition and subtraction of fractions.
2. **Invert** To turn upside down.
3. **Reciprocal** A mathematical term to describe an inverted fraction.
4. **Simplify** A mathematical term used to express the action of reducing fractions to lowest terms.

## ADDING AND SUBTRACTING FRACTIONS WITH COMMON DENOMINATORS

When adding and subtracting fractions, the most important point to remember is that you are actually only **adding or subtracting the _numerators._**

In adding or subtracting fractions, the first step is to make sure the **denominators of all the fractions are alike.** This is known as a _common denominator_.

Let's work with some fractions that have the same or common denominator.

$$\frac{4}{5} + \frac{2}{5} = \frac{6}{5}$$

We added the numerators together and have the common denominators.

Now we need to convert our **improper fraction** to **a mixed number.**

$6 \div 5 = 1\,r\,1$

So our mixed number is $1\frac{1}{5}$.

### EXAMPLE

**Adding** fractions with common denominators.

**STEP 1** Add your numerators.

$$\frac{4}{7} + \frac{2}{7} = \frac{6}{7}$$

**STEP 2** Convert your fraction to a **mixed number** or a **lowest term fraction**.

In this case, our fraction is already in lowest terms, so we are all done!

$$\frac{6}{7}$$

### EXAMPLE

**STEP 1** Add the numerators.

$$\frac{4}{8} + \frac{1}{8} + \frac{10}{8} = \frac{15}{8}$$

**STEP 2** Convert to lowest term and/or a mixed number.

$$15 \div 8 = 1\ r\ 7$$

So our mixed number is $1\frac{7}{8}$.

We use the same process for subtracting fractions. The key is having **like denominators**.

### EXAMPLE

**Subtracting** fractions with common denominators.

**STEP 1** Subtract your **numerators**.

$$\frac{10}{15} - \frac{4}{15} = \frac{6}{15}$$

**STEP 2** Simplify your fraction to the lowest terms. Since both 6 and 15 are divisible by 3, we need to divide to get to the lowest terms.

$$\frac{6 \div 3}{15 \div 3} = \frac{2}{5}$$

**Answer:** $\dfrac{6}{15} = \dfrac{2}{5}$

## Practice Exercise 4-1 Solve the following equations; convert to a mixed number and/or a lowest term fraction.

1. $\dfrac{1}{6} + \dfrac{9}{6} + \dfrac{5}{6} =$ _____

2. $\dfrac{20}{25} + \dfrac{9}{25} =$ _____

3. $\dfrac{3}{10} + \dfrac{4}{10} =$ _____

4. $\dfrac{3}{4} + \dfrac{12}{4} + \dfrac{2}{4} =$ _____

**5.** $\dfrac{2}{11} + \dfrac{6}{11} =$ _____

**8.** $\dfrac{16}{17} - \dfrac{4}{17} =$ _____

**6.** $\dfrac{4}{9} - \dfrac{1}{9} - \dfrac{2}{9} =$ _____

**9.** $\dfrac{39}{94} - \dfrac{9}{94} - \dfrac{11}{94} =$ _____

**7.** $\dfrac{20}{57} - \dfrac{12}{57} =$ _____

**10.** $\dfrac{11}{20} - \dfrac{3}{20} =$ _____

# ADDING AND SUBTRACTING FRACTIONS WITH DIFFERENT DENOMINATORS

What if we are adding or subtracting fractions that have denominators that are different?

$$\frac{4}{7} + \frac{2}{3} = ?$$

We need to find a common denominator. Recall that a common denominator is the number quantity by which all denominators in a set of fractions may be divided evenly.

This is another case where knowing your multiplication tables is necessary.

To find the common denominator, first, we need to find a number that is a multiple of both the denominators of 3 and 7.

$$\frac{4}{7} + \frac{2}{3} = ?$$

Denominators

Both 3 and 7 are multiples of 21, so we need to find the multiple to equal 21 for each denominator.

$$7 \times 3 = 21$$
$$3 \times 7 = 21$$

Our common denominator is 21.

Now, let's continue with our addition problem from the example above.

Because we multiplied the denominators by our multiple of 3 and 7, we **<u>must</u>** also multiply the numerators by the same multiples to ensure we keep the value of our original fractions.

Now we multiply our numerators by the **same** multiples we used to get our new denominator.

Numerators

$$\frac{4}{7} + \frac{2}{3} = ?$$

$$\frac{4 \times 3 = 12}{7 \times 3 = 21} \qquad \frac{4}{7} = \frac{12}{21}$$

$$\frac{2 \times 7 = 14}{3 \times 7 = 21} \qquad \frac{2}{3} = \frac{14}{21}$$

Next, we can set up our addition equation using our **new** *common denominator*.

$$\frac{12}{21} + \frac{14}{21} =$$

Add your numerators.

$$12 + 14 = 26$$

And put it over your denominator to solve the equation.

$$\frac{26}{21}$$

Are we done? No. We need to reduce it to the lowest term or mixed number.

Since our fraction is improper, we need to make it a mixed number.

Divide our numerator by our denominator.

$$26 \div 21 = 1\,r\,5$$

So our mixed number is:

$$1\frac{5}{21}$$

Yah, we did it!

---

### E X A M P L E

**Adding** fractions with different denominators.

$$\frac{5}{6} + \frac{3}{4} = ?$$

**STEP 1** Find **the lowest** multiple of both your denominators (6 and 4).

$$6 \times 2 = 12$$
$$4 \times 3 = 12$$

**STEP 2** Multiply your numerators by the **same** multiple as your denominator.

$$\frac{5 \times 2 = \boxed{10}}{6 \times 2 = \boxed{12}}$$

$$\frac{3 \times 3 = \boxed{9}}{4 \times 3 = \boxed{12}}$$

**STEP 3** Set up your addition equation with the new fractions, and solve.

$$\frac{10}{12} + \frac{9}{12} = \frac{19}{12}$$

**STEP 4** Convert your answer to a mixed number and/or a lowest term fraction.

$$19 \div 12 = 1\,r\,7$$

$$1\frac{7}{12}$$

**STEP 5** Check the fraction in your mixed number to make sure it is in lowest terms.

In this case, there is no number evenly divisible by 7 or 12 (other than 1).

So our fraction *is* in the lowest terms.

18

**Practice Exercise 4-2**  Find the **common denominator** for the following fraction pairs, then add the fractions and reduce to lowest terms when needed.

1. $\dfrac{4}{7}$ and $\dfrac{5}{6}$, _____   $\dfrac{4}{7}+\dfrac{5}{6}=$ _____     4. $\dfrac{2}{3}$ and $\dfrac{5}{7}$, _____   $\dfrac{2}{3}+\dfrac{5}{7}=$ _____

2. $\dfrac{5}{24}$ and $\dfrac{1}{6}$, _____   $\dfrac{5}{24}+\dfrac{1}{6}=$ _____     5. $\dfrac{7}{8}$ and $\dfrac{4}{5}$, _____   $\dfrac{7}{8}+\dfrac{4}{5}=$ _____

3. $\dfrac{5}{9}$ and $\dfrac{2}{27}$, _____   $\dfrac{5}{9}+\dfrac{2}{27}=$ _____

Subtracting fractions with different denominators uses the same concepts.

---

### EXAMPLE

**Subtracting** fractions with different denominators.

$$\frac{17}{18}-\frac{4}{6}=?$$

**STEP 1**  Find a multiple of both the denominators.

In this case we will use 18.

$\dfrac{17}{18}$ already has the correct denominator, so there is no need to change it.

We just need to change our second fraction $\dfrac{4}{6}$.

$6 \times 3 = 18$

**STEP 2**  Multiply your numerator by the **same** multiple as your denominator.

$$\frac{4 \times 3 = 12}{6 \times 3 = 18}$$

**STEP 3**  Set up your subtraction equation and solve.

$$\frac{17}{18}-\frac{12}{18}=\frac{5}{18}$$

**STEP 4**  Convert your fraction to lowest terms or a mixed number.

There is no number evenly divisible by 5 or 18 (besides 1).

Thus our fraction is already in lowest terms.

---

### TIPS FOR SUCCESS

If you are having difficulty finding a common denominator, multiply them!

$$\frac{4}{13}+\frac{3}{8}=$$

$13 \times 8 = 104$ ⟵      *common denominator*

If both the numerator and denominator are **even** numbers, they are divisible by **2**.

If both the numerator and denominator **end in 5**, they are divisible by 5.

This can help you when reducing fractions to lowest terms.

**Practice Exercise 4-3**  Solve the following equations, converting to a mixed number and/or the lowest term fraction.

1. $\dfrac{5}{6} + \dfrac{7}{9} =$  _____

2. $\dfrac{1}{5} + \dfrac{4}{5} + \dfrac{12}{15} =$  _____

3. $\dfrac{3}{8} + \dfrac{15}{16} + \dfrac{1}{2} =$  _____

4. $\dfrac{6}{7} + \dfrac{3}{4} =$  _____

5. $\dfrac{15}{16} + \dfrac{3}{8} + \dfrac{1}{2} =$  _____

6. $\dfrac{13}{33} - \dfrac{1}{11} - \dfrac{2}{11} =$  _____

7. $\dfrac{43}{54} - \dfrac{19}{27} =$  _____

8. $\dfrac{19}{18} - \dfrac{3}{9} - \dfrac{2}{3} =$  _____

9. $\dfrac{15}{6} - \dfrac{2}{3} - \dfrac{1}{2} =$  _____

10. $\dfrac{30}{32} - \dfrac{5}{8} =$  _____

# ADDING OR SUBTRACTING FRACTIONS AND MIXED OR WHOLE NUMBERS

A mixed number or a whole number needs to be converted into a fraction in order to add or subtract it from another fraction.

To turn a whole number into a fraction we simply use the whole number as **both** the numerator and the denominator.

So the whole number six becomes the fraction $\dfrac{6}{1}$.

A mixed number needs to be converted into a fraction as well. Remember that a fraction converted from a mixed number will be improper. This is perfectly fine. After we are done adding or subtracting the fractions together, we will convert it back to a mixed a number.

---

**EXAMPLE**

**Adding** fractions or Whole numbers and Mixed Numbers.

$$\frac{5}{18} + 4\frac{2}{3} + 3 = ?$$

**STEP 1** Convert the mixed number to a fraction.

$$4\frac{2}{3} = \frac{14}{3}$$

**STEP 2** Convert your whole number to a fraction.

$$3 = \frac{3}{1}$$

**STEP 3** Set up your new equation.

$$\frac{5}{18} + \frac{14}{3} + \frac{3}{1} =$$

**STEP 4** Find a common denominator for your fractions. In this case, we use 18.

**STEP 5** Change all your fractions so they have 18 as the denominator. This fraction will stay the same.

$$\boxed{\dfrac{5}{18}}$$

We need to multiply the others as shown below.

$$\dfrac{14 \times 6 = \boxed{84}}{3 \times 6 = \boxed{18}} \qquad\qquad \dfrac{3 \times 18 = \boxed{54}}{1 \times 18 = \boxed{18}}$$

**STEP 6** Set up the equation using our common denominator.

$$\dfrac{5}{18} + \dfrac{84}{18} + \dfrac{54}{18} =$$

**STEP 7** Add the numerators together and show as a fraction over your common denominator.

$$\dfrac{\boxed{5}}{18} + \dfrac{\boxed{84}}{18} + \dfrac{\boxed{54}}{18} = \dfrac{143}{18}$$

**STEP 8** Convert the answer to a mixed number.

$$143 \div 18 = 7\,r\,17$$

**STEP 9** Place the remainder over your new denominator to complete your mixed number.

Remainder

$$\dfrac{107}{18} = 7\dfrac{17}{18}$$

**STEP 10** Make sure your **remainder fraction** is in the lowest terms.

In this case, $7\dfrac{17}{18}$ is the lowest terms.

---

### EXAMPLE

**Subtracting** fractions and Mixed Numbers.

$$3\dfrac{5}{9} - \dfrac{2}{3} - 2 = ?$$

**STEP 1** Convert the mixed number to a fraction.

$$3\dfrac{5}{9} = \dfrac{32}{9}$$

**STEP 2** Convert your whole number to a fraction.

$$2 = \dfrac{2}{1}$$

—Continued next page

*Continued—*

**STEP 3** Set up your new equation.

$$\frac{32}{9} - \frac{2}{3} - \frac{2}{1} =$$

**STEP 4** Find a common denominator for your fractions. In this case we use 18.

**STEP 5** Change all your fractions so they have 18 as the denominator.

$$\frac{32 \times 2 = \boxed{64}}{9 \times 2 = \boxed{18}}$$

$$\frac{2 \times 6 = \boxed{12}}{3 \times 6 = \boxed{18}}$$

$$\frac{2 \times 18 = \boxed{36}}{1 \times 18 = \boxed{18}}$$

**STEP 6** Set up the equation using the common denominator.

$$\frac{64}{18} - \frac{12}{18} - \frac{36}{18} =$$

**STEP 7** **Subtract** the numerators and show your answer as a fraction over your common denominator.

$$\frac{\boxed{64}}{18} - \frac{12}{18} - \frac{36}{18} = \frac{16}{18}$$

**STEP 8** Convert your fraction to the lowest terms.

Both 2 and 18 are divisible by 2.

$$\frac{16 \div 2 = 8}{18 \div 2 = 9}$$

$$\frac{8}{9}$$

Great job!

## Practice Exercise 4-4   Solve the following equations, converting your answer to a mixed number and/or a lowest term fraction.

1. $4\frac{3}{4} - 1\frac{2}{5} =$  _____

2. $1\frac{1}{10} + \frac{7}{12} =$  _____

3. $1\frac{9}{22} - \frac{1}{11} =$  _____

4. $3\frac{1}{8} + \frac{2}{3} + \frac{6}{12} =$  _____

5. $2\frac{4}{13} - \frac{5}{26} =$  _____

6. $\frac{3}{3} + \frac{7}{9} + 5\frac{2}{5} =$  _____

7. $1\frac{3}{8} - \frac{2}{2} =$  _____

8. $5\frac{1}{16} + 1\frac{1}{3} =$  _____

9. $2\frac{19}{21} - \frac{3}{7} =$  _____

10. $1\frac{7}{8} + \frac{2}{13} =$  _____

# MULTIPLYING FRACTIONS AND MIXED NUMBERS

Multiplying fractions is the simplest of the operations we will learn to do with fractions.

All we have to do is multiply our numerators and multiply our denominators. No tricks, no common denominators, just simple multiplication!

Let's try one!

$$\frac{2}{5} \times \frac{4}{8} = ?$$

First we multiply our numerators.

$$2 \times 4 = 8$$

Next, we multiply our denominators.

$$5 \times 8 = 40$$

So our product is $\frac{8}{40}$.

Wow, that was easy! Now we need to simplify our fraction to lowest terms.

$$\frac{8}{40} = \frac{1}{5}$$

What if our equation has a mixed number?

$$5\frac{3}{4} \times \frac{5}{12} = ?$$

Change the mixed number to an improper fraction.

$$5\frac{3}{4} = \frac{23}{4}$$

Then multiply your numerators and denominators.

$$\frac{23}{4} \times \frac{5}{12} = \frac{115}{48}$$

Convert our improper fraction to a mixed number and simplify to the lowest terms.

$$\frac{115}{48} = 2\frac{19}{48}$$

---

**EXAMPLE**

$$2\frac{2}{5} \times \frac{4}{5} = ?$$

**STEP 1** Convert the mixed number to an improper fraction.

$$2\frac{2}{5} = \frac{12}{5}$$

**STEP 2** Multiply the numerators.

$$12 \times 4 = 48$$

**STEP 3** Multiply the denominators.

$$5 \times 5 = 25$$

**STEP 4** Convert the product to a mixed number and a lowest term fraction.

$$\frac{48}{25} = 1\frac{23}{25}$$

**Practice Exercise 4-5**    Solve the following equations, converting your answer to a mixed number and/or a lowest term fraction.

1.  $\dfrac{7}{8} \times \dfrac{5}{13} =$    _____

2.  $2\dfrac{9}{10} \times \dfrac{1}{12} =$    _____

3.  $\dfrac{9}{13} \times 4\dfrac{2}{5} =$    _____

4.  $\dfrac{4}{19} \times 1\dfrac{3}{4} =$    _____

5.  $5\dfrac{5}{8} \times 3\dfrac{4}{13} =$    _____

6.  $\dfrac{16}{17} \times \dfrac{7}{9} =$    _____

7.  $\dfrac{12}{13} \times \dfrac{3}{13} =$    _____

# DIVIDING FRACTIONS AND MIXED NUMBERS

Dividing fractions is basically the same as multiplying fractions with <u>one extra step</u>.

**Always invert your second fraction or the fraction you are "dividing by."** An inverted fraction just means turning the fraction upside down. The denominator becomes the numerator and the numerator becomes the denominator. An inverted or upside-down fraction is known as the *reciprocal*.

Let's look at an example so we get a better understanding.

---

**E X A M P L E**

$\dfrac{4}{5} \div \dfrac{1}{4} = ?$

**STEP 1** Take your second fraction, the fraction you are "dividing by," and **invert** it.

$\dfrac{1}{4}$

**becomes**

$\dfrac{4}{1}$

**STEP 2** Set up your new equation as multiplication.

$\dfrac{4}{5} \times \dfrac{4}{1} =$

**STEP 3** Solve your multiplication equation.

$\dfrac{4}{5} \times \dfrac{4}{1} = \dfrac{16}{5}$

**STEP 4** Simplify your fraction to the lowest terms or a mixed number.

$\dfrac{16}{5} = 3\dfrac{1}{5}$

Dividing mixed numbers works the same way. Just change your mixed numbers to improper fractions and invert the second fraction that you are "dividing by."

We should try one.

## EXAMPLE

$$2\frac{1}{3} \div 4\frac{1}{2} = ?$$

**STEP 1** Change your mixed numbers to improper fractions.

$$\frac{7}{3} \div \frac{9}{2} =$$

**STEP 2** Invert your second or "divided by" fraction.

$$\frac{9}{2}$$

Becomes

$$\frac{2}{9}$$

**STEP 3** Set up the multiplication equation using the reciprocal.

$$\frac{7}{3} \times \frac{2}{9} =$$

**STEP 4** Solve your equation.

$$\frac{7}{3} \times \frac{2}{9} = \frac{14}{27}$$

**STEP 5** Reduce your fraction to lowest terms or a mixed number.

$$\frac{14}{27}$$

This fraction cannot be reduced, so we are finished!

**Practice Exercise 4-6**  Solve the following equations, converting your answer to a mixed number and/or the lowest term fraction.

1. $4\frac{1}{2} \div 2\frac{2}{3} =$ _____

2. $3\frac{3}{5} \div 2\frac{3}{10} =$ _____

3. $\frac{13}{42} \div \frac{4}{5} =$ _____

4. $1\frac{3}{8} \div \frac{1}{8} =$ _____

5. $9\frac{4}{5} \div 2 =$ _____

## Recipes for success......

### SCENARIO 1

Your class is having a fundraiser bake sale. This will benefit the new children' play area at the local hospital.

You decide to make Special Secret Cookies. The recipe makes 120 cookies. Use your subtraction and division skills to figure out how much of each ingredient is needed to make 90 cookies.

### Special Secret Cookies

$\frac{1}{2}$ cup of butter, melted                          _____

$3\frac{1}{2}$ cups sugar                                   _____

3 eggs (beaten)                                              _____

1 can condensed tomato soup ($10\frac{1}{2}$ oz.) (Please answer in ounces) _____

$2\frac{1}{4}$ teaspoons cinnamon                          _____

$2\frac{2}{3}$ teaspoons nutmeg                            _____

2 teaspoons baking soda                                     _____

2 teaspoons salt                                            _____

3 cups raisins                                              _____

$2\frac{1}{2}$ cups chopped nuts                           _____

$4\frac{1}{2}$ cups flour                                  _____

### SCENARIO 2

The bake sale is a great success. Total proceeds are \$324.48. Your class decides to use $\frac{1}{4}$ of the proceeds to purchase children's books.

How much did you spend on books?                            _____

How much of the proceeds are left?                          _____

---

**Nursing and Numbers**

A nurse must be able to quickly assess patient care scenarios and reach for those valuable math skills. Continuing with fractions the nurse will have to count and chart amounts.

Using the same example of "give $\frac{1}{4}$ of the 500 mL solution," the patient consumed less than $\frac{1}{4}$ of the solution. Understanding the value of fractions and being able to quickly count, assess and chart events that may affect the health of the patient can result in positive patient outcomes.

## CHAPTER SUMMARY

- Adding and subtracting fractional equations require a common denominator.
- A common denominator is the number quantity by which all denominators in a set of fractions may be divided evenly.
- Multiply denominators to find a common denominator when adding and subtracting fractions.
- Change mixed numbers to improper fractions in order to solve fractional equations.
- Reduce the answers to fractional equations to mixed numbers and/or lowest terms fractions.
- Multiply numerators and multiply denominators to solve fractional multiplication equations.
- An inverted fraction is known as a reciprocal.
- To invert a fraction, turn it upside down.
- When dividing fractions, invert the second or "divided by" fraction.

## Chapter 4 Practice Test

**Answer *True* or *False* to the following statements:**

1. A reciprocal is a term used to describe an inverted fraction. _____

2. Never use an improper fraction when doing calculations with fractions. _____

3. Adding and subtracting fractions never use a common denominator. _____

4. When dividing fractions, you must use a common denominator. _____

5. To invert a fraction is to turn it upside down. _____

6. A common denominator is a number quantity by which all denominators in a set of fractions may be divided evenly. _____

**Solve the following fraction equations. Reduce your answer to Mixed numbers and/or lowest terms fractions.**

1. $1\frac{3}{17} + 3\frac{1}{5} =$ _____

2. $2\frac{1}{5} \div \frac{3}{16} =$ _____

3. $5\frac{7}{11} \times 3\frac{12}{13} =$ _____

4. $3\frac{5}{6} - \frac{4}{19} =$ _____

5. $7\frac{1}{4} \times 2\frac{2}{5} =$ _____

6. $1\frac{5}{8} \div \frac{9}{10} =$ _____

7. $6\frac{5}{11} - 3\frac{1}{9} =$ _____

8. $\frac{3}{14} + 4\frac{2}{5} =$ _____

9. $1\frac{3}{4} + \frac{9}{11} + \frac{7}{11} =$ _____

10. $1\frac{1}{23} \times 3\frac{7}{10} =$ _____

11. $4\frac{6}{7} \div 2\frac{1}{8} =$ _____

12. $5\frac{2}{21} - \frac{7}{8} =$ _____

13. $4\frac{1}{15} \times \frac{9}{22} =$ _____

14. $6\frac{5}{7} + 1\frac{4}{5} =$ _____

15. $4\frac{7}{17} \div 2\frac{1}{4} =$ _____

16. $7\frac{9}{22} - 4\frac{3}{10} =$ _____

**17.** $2\dfrac{4}{17} \times 3 =$ _____

**18.** $8\dfrac{6}{19} - 1\dfrac{5}{19} =$ _____

**19.** $1\dfrac{9}{10} \div \dfrac{3}{7} =$ _____

**20.** $6\dfrac{4}{9} + 2\dfrac{13}{17} =$ _____

**Solve the Story Problem**

You are working as a pharmacy technician in a research facility. You are asked to combine the results of 3 drug trail research studies and then report the overall results with and without study 3. Study 1 and 2 patients were given the actual drug and study 3 patients were given a placebo (a sugar pill). Study 1 reported that 12 of 15 patients responded well to the drug. Study 2 reported that 56 of 60 patients responded well to the drug. Study 3 showed that 2 of 30 patients responded well to the drug.

1. Report the results of the studies with study 3 included. Write fractions for each study writing the patients who responded well to the drug as the numerator and the total number of patients in the study as the denominator. Find the common denominator, add the 3 fractions together, and reduce to lowest terms. _____

2. Report the results of the studies without study 3 included. Subtract the results from study 3 from your answer to question one. Find the common denominator, add the 3 fractions together, and reduce to lowest terms. _____

# CHAPTER 5 Working with Decimals

## INTRODUCTION

Decimals, like fractions, are basically whole numbers separated into parts. The easiest way to picture a decimal in your mind is to think of the different values of money. Whether you are an RN, medical assistant, LPN, patient care technician, dialysis technician, or pharmacy technician, you will work with decimals in performing dosage calculations and administering or dispensing medications. Likewise, if you are a medical administrative assistant or medical billing specialist working the checkout desk at a busy medical clinic, or a pharmacy technician working the pick-up window in a retail pharmacy, you will be working with decimals.

As a nurse or allied health professional, it is important to understand and accurately perform calculations and rounding with different decimal place values. **Remember to do medical math problems with a calculator to avoid making an error.**

### LEARNING OBJECTIVES

1. Understand and identify place values.
2. Understand and identify the value of a fraction.
3. Understand and identify the value of decimals.
4. Explain the commonality between fractions and decimals.
5. Convert fractions to decimals.
6. Convert decimals to fractions.
7. Rounding decimals to different place values.

### KEY TERMS

1. **Decimals** Any number of parts of a whole number separated using a decimal point.
2. **Rounding** Either increasing or decreasing a number to the next digit based on number place value.

## DECIMALS

A decimal, like a fraction, is any number of parts of a whole number or object. Fractions have a numerator and a denominator, which are separated by a fraction bar. Decimals have whole numbers and/or parts of whole numbers separated with a decimal point (.). Fractions and decimals can be used interchangeably to represent fractional parts of a whole. For example, let's look at the fraction $\frac{1}{2}$ and the decimal 0.50. Both can be used to represent a half of 1.00. The key to working with decimals is to remember that each number written with a decimal point has a different value associated with the placement of the number in relation to the placement of the decimal point. Therefore, it is imperative that your decimal point is always written in the correct place to represent the correct value. Recall that place values of whole numbers, in multiples of ten, were discussed in Chapter 2. Now, let's add place values of fractional decimal values. **Any number written to the left of the decimal point represents a whole number, and any number written to the right of the decimal point represents a fractional decimal value of a whole number.** Here is where money can help with the representation of each place value. For example, twelve dollars and eighty-four cents, $12.84, is written with the whole dollars of 12, to the left of the decimal point $12.84, and the fractional value of 84 cents written to the right of the decimal point $12.**84**. The 84 cents represents a fractional value of only 84 parts of one dollar. Table 5-1 lists the place values used for whole numbers and fractional decimal values in multiples of ten. Let's look at the number 7654.321, notice that **each digit decreases in value as we move from left to right**.

### TABLE 5-1 Place Values

| Whole Numbers | | | | Decimal Point | Fractional Decimal Values | | |
|---|---|---|---|---|---|---|---|
| Thousands | Hundreds | Tens | Ones | . | Tenths | Hundredths | Thousandths |
| 7 | 6 | 5 | 4 | . | 3 | 2 | 1 |

### EXAMPLE

Using Table 5-1, let's determine the place value of each digit in the number 7654.*321*.

Whole numbers written to the left of the decimal place are:

7 is in the **thousands** place = 7 × **1000**

6 is in the **hundreds** place = 6 × **100**

5 is in the **tenths** place = 5 × **10**

4 is in the **ones** place = 4 × **1**

**7654.***321*

Fractional decimal values written to right of the decimal point are:

7654.***321***

*3* is in the **ten<u>ths</u>** place = 3 × **one tenth (1/10)**

*2* is in the **hundred<u>ths</u>** place = 2 × **one hundredth (1/100)**

*1* is in the **thousand<u>ths</u>** place = 1 × **one thousandth (1/1000)**

**Practice Exercise 5-1** Identify the place value for the **bold underlined** numbers.

1. 68**4**3.975 _____
2. 4**9**71.583 _____
3. 8273.64**5** _____
4. **1**029.384 _____
5. 2468.**0**13 _____

6. 837**2**.109 _____
7. 3579.2**4**6 _____
8. 5**9**84.736 _____
9. 7249.**3**58 _____
10. **5**640.713 _____

## CONVERTING FRACTIONS TO DECIMALS

Now that we understand whole and fractional place values, we can convert fractions to decimals. Basically all we are doing in converting from fractions to decimals is changing the way our digits are written. Remember fractions are written with a fraction bar separating the numerator (part) from the denominator (total parts in the whole). An example is $\frac{1}{10}$. When writing fractional decimals, we always use the placeholder of **zero**, and the parts are written in the place value associated with the number of parts represented. Changing $\frac{1}{10}$ to a decimal would be 0.10. When writing mixed numbers in fractions, the whole number is written to the left of the fraction $1\frac{1}{10}$; likewise with writing decimals, the whole number is written to the left of the decimal 1.10. Converting the fraction to a decimal, our answer would be $1\frac{1}{10} = 1.10$.

When you need to determine your fractional decimal value, you divide your numerator by your denominator.

Let's try one!

---

**EXAMPLE**

Convert $1\frac{3}{4}$ to a decimal

**STEP 1** Write the whole number of 1 to the right of the decimal point.

1.

**STEP 2** Determine the fractional decimal value of $\frac{3}{4}$.

Divide the numerator of 3, by the denominator of 4.

$3 \div 4 = 0.75$

**STEP 3** Write your fractional decimal value to the right of the decimal point.

1.**75**

The fraction $1\frac{3}{4}$ converted to a decimal is 1.75.

---

**Practice Exercise 5-2**  Convert the following fractions to decimals.

1. $2\frac{6}{8}$ _____

2. $\frac{1}{4}$ _____

3. $3\frac{3}{5}$ _____

4. $\frac{15}{75}$ _____

5. $4\frac{45}{90}$ _____

## CONVERTING DECIMALS TO FRACTIONS

Converting decimals to fractions is just as easy as converting fractions to decimals. Here we rewrite the decimal as a fraction over the place value of the fractional decimal and reduce to the lowest terms. Recall that reducing to the lowest terms was discussed in chapter 3. Let's look at the decimal answer from the example in the previous section of 1.75. We need to determine the place value of 0.75. To do this, you always use the value of the **digit farthest to the right of the decimal point**. In this case, the 5, which is the farthest digit to the right, is in the hundredths place. Our fractional decimal value of 0.75 can be rewritten as the fraction of $\frac{75}{100}$.

Let's try it!

---

**EXAMPLE**

Convert the decimal 1.75 to a fraction.

**STEP 1** Write the whole number to the left of the fraction.

1—

**STEP 2** Determine the fractional value of the fractional decimal, and write a fraction.

0.7**5**

The 5 is in the hundredths value place.

$0.75 = \frac{75}{100}$

**STEP 3** Write the fraction to the right of the whole number, and reduce to lowest terms.

$1\frac{75}{100} = 1\frac{3}{4}$

---

**Practice Exercise 5-3**  Convert the following decimals to fractions or mixed numbers.

1. 6.75 _____          4. 1.70 _____

2. .5 _____            5. 3.30 _____

3. .25 _____

# ROUNDING

When working with decimals, you may have to round your answers to the nearest fractional value of tenths, hundredths, or thousandths, especially if you use a calculator. The answer on the calculator may repeat and be displayed in multiple decimal places. For example, you are converting from a fraction to a decimal. The fraction is $\frac{1}{3}$, so you divide 1 by 3 and your calculator displays the answer as 0.33333... Your original fractional value of $\frac{1}{3}$ is in tenths; therefore, you need to round your calculator answer to the tenths place value. The answer is $\frac{1}{3}$ = 0.3. There two are rules for rounding that you must follow when working with decimals in order to get the correct answer.

## Rules for Rounding

### Rule 1

If the number to the right of the desired place value is 1 through 4, do not change the value of the number. **This is called rounding down.**

**48.12 = 48.1**

### Rule 2

If the number to the right of the desired place value is 5 through 9, round by adding 1 to the value in the desired place value. **This is called rounding up.**

**25.56 = 25.6**

**Practice Exercise 5-4**  Round to the nearest, tenths or hundredths.

1. 1.473 _____         4. 0.141 _____

2. 0.192 _____         5. 1.789 _____

3. 3.051 _____

## MANUAL MATH CORNER

Remember you may have to ***manually*** round decimals.

Practice identifying your place values and recalling your rounding rules.

7654.*321* Numbers to the left of the decimal are whole numbers and numbers to the right of the decimal are fractional parts (decimals).

0, 1, 2, 3, 4... round down

5, 6, 7, 8, 9... round up

## Recipes for success......

### SCENARIO 1

It is time for the annual company picnic. They are giving a prize of $250.00 to the best barbecue sauce recipe. Uncle Charlie has won several barbecue competitions and agrees to help you create a great sauce. You agree to give him half the prize money if you win.

*Convert the following recipe to decimals, round your answer if needed.*

### The Absolute Best Barbecue Sauce

$2\frac{1}{4}$ teaspoons vinegar _____

$1\frac{1}{2}$ teaspoons salt _____

$1\frac{3}{4}$ teaspoons pepper _____

$\frac{2}{3}$ cup of honey _____

$3\frac{2}{3}$ cups of ketchup _____

$2\frac{1}{3}$ cloves of garlic (finely chopped) _____

$\frac{1}{4}$ cup molasses _____

$\frac{5}{6}$ teaspoons of Dijon style mustard _____

### SCENARIO 2

Uncle Charlie's recipe wins the contest! You both decide to split the prize money among your favorite charities. Three organizations are chosen. How much of the total will each charitable organization get? Round your dollar amount if needed. _____

---

**Nursing and Numbers**

Converting from fractions to decimals will occur in nursing care.

You may have to give $\frac{1}{2}$ of a dose of medication and the dose is given in decimals. An example would be the medication only is available in 0.75 mg. Reach for your math skills and convert to the decimal dose.

---

## CHAPTER SUMMARY

- A decimal is any number of parts of a whole number separated using a decimal point.
- Fractions and decimals can be used interchangeably to represent fractional parts of a whole.
- Any number written to the *left* of the decimal point represents a whole number.
- Any number written to the *right* of the decimal point represents a fractional decimal value.
- To determine a fractional decimal value, divide your numerator by your denominator.
- A decimal can be converted to a fraction by rewriting the decimal over the place value of the fractional decimal and reduce to the lowest terms.
- If the number to the right of the desired place value is 1 through 4, do not change the value of the number (round down).
- If the number to the right of the desired place value is 5 through 9, round by adding 1 to the value in the desired place value (round up).

## Chapter 5 Practice Test

**Answer *True* or *False* to the following statements:**

1. A number *right* of the decimal point is a fractional value. _____

2. There are four rules for rounding. _____

3. To determine the place value of 0.45, use the value of the digit farthest to the *left* of the decimal point. _____

4. Numbers to the *left* of the decimal are whole numbers. _____

5. Understanding place values is an important concept when working with decimals. _____

6. If the number to the *right* of the desired place value is 1 through 4, you will need to round up. _____

**Identify the place value for the bold underlined numbers.**

1. 901**6**.158 _____
2. 5839.2**7**9 _____
3. 4**9**05.376 _____
4. 9872.**3**58 _____
5. **4**650.931 _____

6. 5743.**6**83 _____
7. 7**9**14.835 _____
8. 6**3**54.725 _____
9. **1**948.214 _____
10. 2468.**3**13 _____

**Convert the following Fractions to Decimals; round to the appropriate place value when needed.**

1. $3\frac{2}{12}$ _____
2. $\frac{2}{5}$ _____
3. $7\frac{6}{8}$ _____
4. $1\frac{12}{13}$ _____
5. $4\frac{3}{9}$ _____

6. $\frac{6}{12}$ _____
7. $2\frac{4}{19}$ _____
8. $5\frac{2}{3}$ _____
9. $3\frac{12}{16}$ _____
10. $5\frac{1}{5}$ _____

**Convert the following Decimals to Fractions; reduce to lowest terms when needed.**

1. 4.25 _____
2. 7.5 _____
3. 1.2 _____
4. 0.75 _____
5. 9.05 _____

6. 2.5 _____
7. 0.8 _____
8. 1.25 _____
9. 6.4 _____
10. 0.025 _____

**Solve the Story Problem**

You are a medical assistant working in a pediatric practice located in the north tower of the professional building adjacent to the Regional Children's Medical Center. Each day is broken into two 3-hour blocks of time for scheduling patients, 9:00 a.m. to 12:00 p.m. and 1:00 p.m. to 4:00 p.m. The providers and physicians have a weekly 3-hour practice meeting on Wednesday afternoons; therefore, no patients are scheduled for the second half of the day. During the provider practice meeting, the Office Manager has a 1-hour staff meeting. After the staff meeting, the patient examination rooms, reception areas, and the waiting rooms are stocked with supplies. This is followed with a weekly inventory of each department. The practice has 6 examination rooms and 4 waiting rooms. The waiting rooms include 1 main waiting room, 2 infectious child waiting rooms, and a postprocedure waiting room.

1. Practice meetings are held for 3 hours every Wednesday afternoon. What portion of the scheduling day is not available for scheduling patients? Write your answer in a fraction and then convert it to a decimal. _____

2. The practice has 6 examination rooms and 4 waiting rooms. The total number of patient rooms is 10. Write a fraction with the examination rooms as the numerator and total number of patient rooms as the denominator. Convert your answer to a decimal, round when needed. _____

3. During the medical practice 3-hour meeting, you attend a 1-hour staff meeting. How many hours are spent stocking rooms and taking inventory? Write a fraction with your answer of time spent stocking rooms and doing inventory as the numerator and the total hours of the medical practice meeting as the denominator. Convert your answer to a decimal, round when needed. _____

4. The practice has 4 waiting rooms. Two of the waiting rooms are for sick children, 1 is a postprocedure waiting room, and 1 is a main waiting room. Write a fraction for each of the types of waiting rooms, with the type of waiting room as the numerator and the total number of waiting rooms as the denominator. Convert your answers to decimals.

Sick waiting rooms _____

Postprocedure waiting room _____

Main waiting room _____

# 6 Basic Operations with Decimals

## INTRODUCTION

Basic addition, subtraction, multiplication, and division of decimals are skills that are used in every facet of allied health and nursing. A complete knowledge and ability to do these types of mathematical calculations are imperative to any health profession. The incorrect placement of the decimal point can lead to serious or even deadly consequences to a patient. Remember to always use a calculator for medical math calculations, and double check your work. If there is any doubt in your mind that the math problem has been set up or done incorrectly ask another health professional to check the math to ensure correctness.

### KEY TERMS

1. **Divisor** A mathematical term to describe the number "*divided by.*"
2. **Dividend** A mathematical term to describe the number "*that is being divided.*"

## ADDING AND SUBTRACTING DECIMALS

Adding and subtracting decimals are very similar to that of whole numbers. The most important thing to understand and remember is that **all numbers have a place value**.

When adding or subtracting decimals you need to make sure that the decimal point lines up in the same place throughout the problem.

Let's try a few.

$$143.67 + 74.8 = ?$$

The easiest way to make sure the decimal points line up is to stack the equation, just like we did with the whole numbers in chapter 2.

```
  143.67
+  74.8
```

In this equation, there are two places **after** the decimal point in our first number.

We can add a zero as a place holder **after** the 8 to help us line things up correctly.

```
  143.67
+  74.80  ⟵
```

We confirm that our decimal points are lined up directly beneath one another to ensure our place values are correct.

Now we can solve our equation.

$$143.67$$
$$+\ 74.80$$
$$218.47$$

Now try a subtraction equation.

$$213.09 - 43.908 = ?$$

Just like in addition, we need to stack the equation so we can line up the decimal points.

$$213.09$$
$$-\ 43.908$$

We can add a zero as a place holder after the 9 in our first decimal to help us line up our numbers.

$$213.090 \longleftarrow$$
$$-\ 43.908$$

Now solve the equation.

$$213.090$$
$$-\ 43.908$$
$$169.182$$

## TIPS FOR SUCCESS...

When adding or subtracting decimals, the decimal points need to line up.

Remember that the decimal point always goes to the **right** of the ones place.

Recall from Chapter 2 to always start with the number furthest to the right and work left.

Remember to use the "**carry over method**" when your numbers add up to ten or more.

Remember to use the "**borrowing method**" if the digit being subtracted in a column is larger than the digit above it.

One more time to make sure we understand.

### EXAMPLE

**Adding** decimals.

$$42.053 + 180.61 = ?$$

**STEP 1** Stack the numbers so they are easy to line up.

$$42.053$$
$$+180.61$$

**STEP 2** Make sure the decimal points line up throughout the problem. In this problem, there are digits **three places to the left of the decimal point**. This should be the same in our answer.

$$42.053$$
$$+180.61$$

**STEP 3** Add a zero in the *thousandths* place after the decimal point to ensure the decimals line up correctly.

$$42.053$$
$$+180.610 \longleftarrow$$

**STEP 4** Solve the equation

```
   42.053
+ 180.610
  222.663  ⟵
```

Notice we have three places used after the decimal point.

**Subtracting** decimals.

$156.29 - 38.431 = ?$

**STEP 1** Stack the numbers so they are easier to line up.

```
  156.29
-  38.431
```

**STEP 2** Make sure the decimal points line up throughout the problem. In this problem, there are digits **three places to the left of the decimal point**. This should be the same in our answer.

**STEP 3** Add a zero in the *thousandths* place after the decimal point to ensure the decimals line up correctly.

```
  156.290  ⟵
-  38.431
```

**STEP 4** Solve the equation

```
  156.290
-  38.431
  117.859  ⟵
```

Notice we have three places used after the decimal point.

**Practice Exercise 6-1**  Add or subtract the following decimal equations.

1.  255.09
    + 54.8

2.  389.2
    − 122.08

3.  42.240
    +39.06

4.  801.006
    −773.01

5.  92.50
    − 25.101

6.  855.123
    + 66.94

7.  186.742
    − 25.101

8.  255.09
    + 54.8

9.  389.32
    − 122.08

10. 42.240
    + 39.06

## MULTIPLYING AND DIVIDING DECIMALS

**Multiplying decimals** is the simplest of the decimal operations. It does not involve making sure the decimal points line up. Just do the multiplication as if it was all whole numbers. We can ignore our decimals points until we have completed the multiplication.

Let's solve one in order to better understand.

$$42.09 \times .73 = ?$$

Just pretend there are no decimal points, and they are both whole numbers.

$$4209 \times 73 = ?$$

Now solve the equation just like we learned in chapter two.

$$
\begin{array}{r}
4209 \\
\times\ 73 \\
\hline
12627 \\
+\ 294630 \\
\hline
307257
\end{array}
$$

Now we can put in our decimal point.

To do this, count the places to the *right* of the decimal point in both the numbers.

$$42.\boxed{09} \times .\boxed{73}$$

2 + 2 = 4 decimal places

In this case, there are **two** places to the right of the decimal point in the first number, and **two** places to the right of the decimal point in the second number. Our total number of decimal places is **four**.

Take the product from the whole number equation and **count four places, moving from right to left**, and insert the decimal point.

$$30.\boxed{7257}$$

$$42.09 \times .73 = 30.7257$$

We did it!

**Division with decimals** is a little more difficult. It is easier to explain during the process, so let's just get started with an equation.

$$79.221 \div .55 = ?$$

The number you are "dividing by" (.55) is called the *divisor*.

The number you are dividing (79.221) is called the *dividend*.

First turn your divisor into a whole number by moving your decimal point to the right. In this case we are moving the decimal point two places.

.55 *moving **two** decimal places to the **right** becomes* 55.

Next we move the decimal point in our dividend (the number we are dividing) the same amount of places to the right we moved in the divisor. We need to move **two** decimal places to the right.

79.221 *moving **two** decimal places to the **right** becomes* 7922.1.

Now we can do the division equation.

Line up the decimal point in the quotient directly above the decimal point in the dividend.

$$
\begin{array}{r}
144.0381 \\
55.\overline{)7922.1}
\end{array}
$$

Recall from the division we learned in chapter 2, if the problem did not come out evenly, we could complete the equation by writing a remainder. In division with decimals we cannot have a remainder. Because decimals can go on forever, the best way to finish the problem is to use the rounding method we learned in the last chapter.

In this case, let's round the quotient to the *hundredths* place. Use the rules for rounding that were discussed in chapter five.

144.0381 *rounded to the hundreths place becomes* 144.04

## TIPS FOR SUCCESS...

When multiplying decimals, always count from the right and move left when counting decimal places for your product.

When dividing decimals, round your answer; there is no such thing as a remainder in a division decimal equation.

Let's try one more of each.

## EXAMPLE

**Multiplying** decimals.

$67.7 \times 3.81 = ?$

**STEP 1** Pretend there are no decimal points and solve as if multiplying whole numbers.

$677 \times 381 = 257937$

**STEP 2** Count the total places to the right of the decimal point in both numbers of the original equation.

$$67\boxed{7} \times 3\boxed{81} =$$

1  +  2 = 3 decimal places

There are a total of three places to the right of the decimal point.

**STEP 3** Starting with the digit farthest to the right in the product, count three places to the left and add the decimal point.

257.937     Great Job!

## EXAMPLE

**Dividing** decimals:

$10.4 \div 2.4 = ?$

**STEP 1** Move the decimal point in the divisor to the right until it becomes a whole number.

$10.4 \div 24. = ?$

**STEP 2** Move the decimal point in the dividend the same amount of places to the right as the divisor.

$104. \div 24. = ?$

**STEP 3** Solve the equation.

Line up the decimal point in the same place as the decimal point in the dividend.

$$\overset{4.33}{24.\overline{)104.00}}$$

**STEP 4** Round your answer if needed.

### Practice Exercise 6-2    Solve the following equations, round to the nearest hundredths place.

1. $43.27 \times 3.13 =$

2. $199.52 \div 5.2 =$

3. $8.74 \times 8.23 =$

4. $96.159 \div .87 =$

5. $52.18 \times 7.3 =$

6. $41.3 \div 7.021 =$

7. $64.104 \times .12 =$

8. $8.52 \div 1.33 =$

9. $2 \times .691 =$

10. $52.23 \div 7.2 =$

## Recipes for success......

**SCENARIO 1**

You are hosting a party to celebrate your cousin's graduation from practical nursing school. *For dessert, you decide on a "Make Your Own Ice Cream Sunday Bar."*

**Below is a list of the supplies you will need to purchase.**

**Toppings**

| | |
|---|---|
| Strawberry topping | $2.89 per 2 lb container |
| Chocolate syrup | $4.27 per 3 lb bottle |
| Hot fudge | $7.50 per container |
| Candy sprinkles | $2.35 per package |
| Crushed peanuts | $8.54 per 3 lb package |
| Pineapple topping | $4.44 per 18 oz. container |
| Ice cream | $3.79 per gallon |
| Disposable bowls | $9.00 per package of 300 each |
| Disposable spoons | $0.99 per package of 32 each |
| Paper napkins | $1.49 per package of 48 each |

*The ice cream is also available in 5-gallon containers for $16.78 each.*

1. Are the 5-gallon containers of ice cream a better deal if you need to purchase 15 gallons total? _____

2. What is the price per gallon of ice cream in a 5-gallon container? _____

3. What is the total price for 15 gallons of ice cream when buying 5-gallon containers? _____

4. What are your total savings for 15 gallons of ice cream when buying 5-gallon containers? _____

5. What is the cost of 5 lbs. of crushed peanuts? _____

**6.** What is the price per spoon? _____

**7.** What is the total price for 300 spoons? _____

**8.** How many packages of spoons do you need to purchase? _____

**9.** If you need 3 packages/containers of each topping, what would the total cost be?
_____

## SCENARIO 2

Your office is having a potluck luncheon for the physician in charge of your clinic. He received the Physician of the Year award at the Regional Medical Center that your office is affiliated with. There are 12 people working at your clinic. You are asked to bring cucumber finger sandwiches and to make enough for each person to have 2 sandwiches. You need to make 24 cucumber sandwiches. Your recipe is for 48 sandwiches.

*Determine how much of each ingredient you will need to make 24 cucumber sandwiches.*

### Ingredients

4 cucumbers (sliced into 24 slices each)    _____

8 oz. onion and chive-flavored cream cheese spread _____

½ cup ranch salad dressing    _____

¼ teaspoon garlic powder    _____

¼ teaspoon fresh cracked black pepper    _____

1 teaspoon fresh chopped parsley    _____

1 teaspoon fresh minced dill sprigs    _____

48 slices of multigrain bread    _____

Petite round cookie cutter    _____

---

**Nursing and Numbers**

Decimal point placement is crucial. Medical errors because of misuse of decimal points can happen easily. Always recheck your work.

"0" to the left of the decimal point is ALWAYS necessary.

Example:

0.5 not .5

When written incorrectly a medication can be 10 times more than ordered.

Example:

5 instead of 0.5

"0" to the right of the last digit in a decimal should NEVER be used.

Example:

1.2 is correct not 1.20

As you can see the absolute need for correct decimal placement, and the use of the "0" to the left of the decimal point.

## CHAPTER SUMMARY

- Stacking addition and subtraction problems with decimals assist in lining up the decimal points.
- When adding and subtracting decimal equations, the decimal points need to line up directly above and below each other.
- The decimal point always goes to the right of the ones place.
- Use the "carry over or borrowing" method when adding or subtracting decimals, just like with whole numbers.
- When multiplying decimals, count the places to the right of the decimal point and apply to the product of the equation.
- When counting decimal places in the product of a decimal multiplication equation, start from the right and move left.
- Always start from the farthest right digit and move left to solve any decimal equation.
- When dividing decimals, move the decimal point in the divisor to the right until it becomes a whole number.
- When dividing decimals, move the decimal point in the dividend the same amount of places to the right as the divisor.
- The decimal point in a division quotient should be in the same place as the decimal point in the divisor.
- Division quotients do not have remainders.
- Division quotients should be rounded.

## Chapter 6 Practice Test

Answer *True* or *False* to the following statements:

1. The quotient in a decimal division equation allows a remainder. _____

2. Decimal points are not important in the medical setting. _____

3. Always line up the decimal points in an addition or subtraction equation. _____

4. Stacking addition and subtraction decimal problems aid in correctly lining up the decimal points. _____

5. Count the total places to the left of the decimal point in a multiplication product. _____

**Add and Subtract.**

1. $\begin{array}{r} 67.43 \\ +92.4 \\ \hline \end{array}$

2. $\begin{array}{r} 271.05 \\ -\ 87.35 \\ \hline \end{array}$

3. $\begin{array}{r} 42.62 \\ +21.88 \\ \hline \end{array}$

4. $\begin{array}{r} 199.36 \\ -\ \ 8.9 \\ \hline \end{array}$

5. $\begin{array}{r} 592.637 \\ +\ 81.02 \\ \hline \end{array}$

6. $\begin{array}{r} 221.221 \\ -\ 99.999 \\ \hline \end{array}$

7. $\begin{array}{r} 2.538 \\ +889.75 \\ \hline \end{array}$

8. $\begin{array}{r} 79.78 \\ -78.79 \\ \hline \end{array}$

9. $\begin{array}{r} 90.003 \\ +\ 8.61 \\ \hline \end{array}$

10. $\begin{array}{r} 47.69 \\ -23.987 \\ \hline \end{array}$

**Multiply and Divide (*round your answer to the nearest tenth*).**

1. $95.2 \times 18.5 =$

2. $67.987 \div 4.222 =$

3. $152.3 \times .065 =$

4. $84.90 \div 21.7 =$

5. $456.1 \times .188 =$

6. $764.32 \div 84.13 =$

7. $.333 \times 71.21 =$

8. $6.33 \div 1.964 =$

9. $53.1 \times 2.621 =$

10. $995.3 \div 2.75 =$

**Solve the Story Problem**

Your office manager is taking up a collection for a gift to present to the physician in charge. The luncheon is honoring his award as Physician of the Year. She realizes everyone is already contributing to the luncheon by providing food items for the occasion and does not want to put a required dollar amount to donate toward the gift. She decides to start an envelope with money from petty cash. This way, people will be able to make change as well as to ensure no one knows how much each staff member donated. She is starting with the following from petty cash: 3-$10s, 3-$5s, 3-$1s, 6-quarters, 4-dimes, and 2 nickels. The envelope makes it around the office and is returned to the office manager. The total amount in the envelope is $167.40. The office manager needs to take out the money used to start the envelope and return it to the petty cash fund; the remaining amount will be used to purchase the gift. The office manager plans to order a plague honoring the physician. The plaque will hang in the patient waiting room. The plaque costs $75.00. She also plans to buy plastic champagne flutes and alcohol-free bubbling cider for the toast at the luncheon. Plastic champagne flutes are 4.99 for a package of 8 and bubbling cider is $5.75 a bottle. Any remaining money will be used to buy wrapping paper, and a card for all the staff to sign.

1. How much money was used from petty cash to start the envelope? _____

2. How much money is left after paying back the petty cash fund? _____

3. How much will 2 packages of plastic champagne flutes cost? _____

4. How much will 2 bottles of alcohol-free bubbling cider cost? _____

5. How much money is left to use to buy wrapping paper and a card? _____

# 7 Percents, Ratios, and Proportions

## INTRODUCTION

Like fractions and decimals, percents and ratios represent a portion of a whole. The easiest way to picture a percent in your mind is to think of the number 100. A percent is always related to 100 as in 100%. Ratios basically compare two values. You can think of a ratio as having to work 5 out of 7 days a week. You are working a portion of the whole week. Proportions are simply statements that show two ratios are equal and can be very useful when working as a nurse or allied health professional. The last topic we will cover in this chapter is cross multiplication, which is nothing more than working multiplication selecting specific values.

As a nurse or allied health professional, it is important to understand and accurately work with percents, ratios, and proportions. **Remember to do medical math problems with a calculator to avoid making an error.**

## LEARNING OBJECTIVES

1. Explain the commonality between percents, ratios, fractions, and decimals.
2. Convert between percents, ratios, fractions, and decimals.
3. Understand fraction and ratio proportions.
4. Perform cross multiplication to solve for an unknown value.

## KEY TERMS

1. **Cross Multiplication** A mathematical method in which a numerator of a fraction is multiplied by the denominator of another fraction.
2. **Percent** Any amount that is a part of 100.
3. **Proportion** A mathematical term referring to two equal fractions or ratios.
4. **Ratio** A mathematical statement of how two numbers compare. How much of one item or number as compared to another item or number.

## CONVERTING DECIMALS AND PERCENTS

A decimal, like a percent, is any number of parts of a whole number. Decimals and percents can be easily converted. Recall from chapter 5 the fraction $\frac{1}{2}$ and the decimal 0.5. Both can be used to represent a half of 100. Also recall when working with decimals that each number written with a decimal point has a different value associated with the placement of the number in relation to the placement of the decimal point. Now that we reviewed a bit let's add to what you have learned. Take the decimal 0.5 and let's convert it to a percent. **Percentages are always related to the number 100**. To convert a decimal to a percent, we simply **multiply by 100** and add the percentage symbol (%).

> ### EXAMPLE
>
> Convert the decimal 0.5 to a percent.
>
> Multiply 0.5 by 100
> $0.5 \times 100 = 50$
>
> Add the percentage symbol
>
> $0.5 \times 100 = 50\%$
> $0.50 = 50\%$

Let's do one more to make sure we have it perfected.

> ### EXAMPLE
>
> Convert the decimal 1.75 to a percent.
>
> Multiply 1.75 by 100
> $1.75 \times 100 = 175$
>
> Add the percentage symbol
>
> $1.75 \times 100 = 175\%$
> $1.75 = 175\%$

**Practice Exercise 7-1**   Convert the decimals to percents.

**1.** 3.97 _____          **4.** 0.33 _____

**2.** 0.83 _____          **5.** 1.5 _____

**3.** 0.05 _____

Now let's convert a percent to a decimal. Here you **divide by 100** and remove your percentage symbol.

> ### EXAMPLE
>
> Convert 50% to a decimal.
>
> Divide 50% by 100, and remove the percent symbol
> $50\% \div 100 = 0.5$

**Practice Exercise 7-2**   Convert the percents to decimals.

**1.** 75% _____          **4.** 25% _____

**2.** 112% _____         **5.** 3% _____

**3.** 246% _____

## RATIOS AND PROPORTIONS

Working with ratios and proportions is not complicated and actually can be quite fun. A ratio is just like a fraction, decimal, or percent, in that it represents the parts of a whole. The difference is in how we write and read them. Fractions are written with a fraction bar (—), (decimals are written with a decimal point (.), percents are written with the percentage symbol (%), and ratios are written with a colon (:).

When reading a ratio, the colon is read as "is to," so with the ratio 1:2, we would say "one is to two." This is important to remember because we will use it again when we work with proportions. Ratios, like fractions, should be reduced to lowest terms whenever possible. But for now, we will focus on learning to write ratios. We will work with reducing in the next section with working proportions.

Let's write some ratios!

### EXAMPLE

Using the sentence in the chapter introduction, let's write that you work 5 days out of the week as a ratio.

You work 5 days a week (part of the week) and there are 7 days in a week (a whole week).

Our ratio is written as 5:7

Which is read as 5 is to 7.

Let's try writing a fraction as a ratio.

### EXAMPLE

Write the fraction $\frac{1}{2}$ as a ratio

Our ratio is 1:2.

Which is read as 1 is to 2.

Let's write a mixed number as a ratio. To do this, we have to convert the mixed number to an improper fraction.

### EXAMPLE

Write $1\frac{1}{3}$ as a ratio

Convert $1\frac{1}{3}$ to an improper fraction

$1 \times 3 = 3 + 1 = 4$

$1\frac{1}{3} = \frac{4}{3}$

Our ratio is 4:3.

Which is read as 4 is to 3.

We can also write decimals as ratios, to do this we need to convert the decimal to a fraction.

### EXAMPLE

Write 0.25 as a ratio

The number farthest to the right is in the hundredths place, so we know to write our fraction as $\frac{25}{100}$.

Our ratio is 25:100.

Which is read as 25 is to 100.

We can also write percents as ratios. Since we know percents always work with the number 100, all we have to do is write the percent value to the left of the colon and 100 to the right of the colon.

---

**EXAMPLE**

Write 17% as a ratio

Our ratio is 17:100.

Which is read as 17 is to 100.

---

**Practice Exercise 7-3**  Write the following as ratios.

**1.** You work 8 hours a day  _____      **4.** 0.5      _____

**2.** $\frac{2}{7}$      _____      **5.** 75%      _____

**3.** $1\frac{3}{4}$      _____

# PROPORTIONS

Proportions are used to write mathematical statements for two sets of numbers that have the same value (are equal). Working with ratios, just like working with fractions, we want to reduce to lowest terms whenever possible. We can use reducing as an example for writing proportions. For example, the fraction $\frac{25}{100}$ has the same value as the fraction $\frac{1}{4}$ which can be written as a fraction proportion. Our fraction proportion is $\frac{25}{100} = \frac{1}{4}$. When writing ratio proportions we use a double colon (::) between two ratios which is read as the word "as." Using our same numbers, our ratio proportion is 25 : 100 :: 1 : 4, which reads as "25 is to 100 as 1 is to 4."

Our ratio proportion is 25 : 100 :: 1 : 4
Which is read as 25 is to 100 as 1 is to 4.

Let's write a fraction proportion!

---

**EXAMPLE**

Reduce the fraction $\frac{3}{9}$, and write a fraction proportion

$\frac{3}{9}$    reduces to    $\frac{1}{3}$

Our fraction proportion is

$\frac{3}{9} = \frac{1}{3}$

---

Now let's write a ratio proportion

---

**EXAMPLE**

Reduce the ratio 3:9, and write a ratio proportion

3:9 reduces to 1:3

Our ratio proportion is

3 : 9 :: 1 : 3

**Practice Exercise 7-4** Reduce the fraction or ratio to lowest terms; write your answers as proportions.

1. $75 : 100$ _____

2. $\dfrac{50}{100}$ _____

3. $15 : 45$ _____

4. $\dfrac{12}{144}$ _____

5. $8 : 24$ _____

# CROSS MULTIPLICATION

Cross multiplication is commonly used to find unknown values in proportions. Using our previous example of $\dfrac{25}{100} = \dfrac{1}{4}$, let's set up a cross-multiplication equation with an unknown value.

$$\frac{25}{100} = \frac{1}{?}$$

To solve for the missing value we cross multiply. Think of this as the multiplication symbol ×, with arrows.

$$\frac{25}{100} \bowtie \frac{1}{?}$$

Set up and work your cross-multiplication equation

$$25 \times ? = 100 \times 1$$

Since we know both sides of the original proportion are equal, we know that

$$100 \times 1 = 100 \quad \text{and} \quad 25 \times ? = 100$$

To solve for our unknown, we simply divide both sides of our unknown equation by 25. 25 is associated with our unknown value in the cross multiplication equation of $25 \times ?$. We always divided both sides of the cross multiplication equations by the number associated with the unknown value (recall that division can be written as fractions).

$$\frac{25 \times ?}{25} = \frac{100}{25}$$

or

$$25 \div 25 = ? \quad \text{and} \quad 100 \div 25 = 4$$

$$? = 4$$

Let's try one!

---

### EXAMPLE

Using cross multiplication, solve for the unknown value

$$\frac{2}{3} = \frac{4}{?}$$

Set up and work cross multiplication

$$\frac{2}{3} \bowtie \frac{4}{?}$$

$$3 \times 4 = 12 \quad \text{and} \quad 2 \times ? = 12$$

*—Continued next page*

*Continued—*

Divide both sides of the equation by 2

$$\frac{2 \times ?}{2} = \frac{12}{2}$$

or

$$2 \div 2 = ? \quad \text{and} \quad 12 \div 2 = 6$$

$$? = 6$$

**Practice Exercise 7-5** Using cross multiplication, solve for the unknown value.

1. $\frac{5}{25} = \frac{1}{?}$ _____

2. $\frac{?}{36} = \frac{1}{2}$ _____

3. $\frac{9}{12} = \frac{?}{4}$ _____

4. $\frac{?}{45} = \frac{3}{5}$ _____

5. $\frac{3}{7} = \frac{9}{?}$ _____

## MANUAL MATH CORNER

Working with converting decimals and percents can be done manually with ease. Since there are 2 zeros in 100, you simply move your decimal point two places.

**Example:**

You can convert 0.47 to a percent by moving your decimal point two places to the **right** and add the percent symbol.

2 decimal places to the right

$$0.47 = 47\%$$

You can convert 47% (percent) to a decimal by moving your decimal point two places to the **left** and remove the percentage symbol.

2 decimal places to the left

$$47\% = 0.47$$

**Tip:** When you move to the left, the percentage symbol also left (was removed).

## Recipes for success......

### SCENARIO 1

Your medical office volunteers to host a pancake breakfast for wounded veterans in the community. Two colleagues and you are in charge of purchasing the food. To save cash, you and your associates skim the grocery ads for sales and coupons on the items you need.

Attendance is expected to be about 50 adults, including your staff. As a cushion to make sure you have enough food, a staff member suggested adding 15% to your total attendance numbers.

What is the total number of guests expected with the added 15%? (round your answer). _____

You need 6.5 lbs. of flour to make all the pancakes. The flour only comes in 5-lb bags. You will need to buy 2–5-lb bags, giving you a total of 10 lbs. of flour. What percentage of the flour will NOT be used? _____

If the flour costs $3.47 per 5-lb bag and you are getting a 12% discount on each bag, what is the total cost of all the flour? _____

Turkey sausage links are $6.30 for a package containing 20. If each guest has three sausages, how many total packages of sausage do you need to purchase? _____

Write a ratio of total guests to total sausage. _____

What is the total price on the sausage you need to purchase? _____

If you have a coupon for $1.00 off each package of sausage, what is the percentage off each package? _____

**SCENARIO 2**

## Banana Nut Pancakes

*Rewrite each ingredient as a decimal; include the units of measurement (i.e. cups, teaspoon, etc...).*

2½ cups flour              _____

½ cup sugar               _____

½ teaspoon baking soda   _____

¼ teaspoon salt           _____

2 eggs                    _____

1 cup walnuts             _____

2 bananas                 _____

⅔ cup butter             _____

1 cup powdered sugar      _____

---

**Nursing and Numbers**

The nurse has to make patient serum to be used in an allergist's office. The use of ratios is needed because each patient has a specific serum for their allergy needs. Mixing the allergy serum will be calculated with portions of the whole using ratios.

---

## CHAPTER SUMMARY

- A decimal, like a percent, is any number of parts of a whole number.
- Each number written with a decimal point has a different value associated with the placement of the number.
- To convert a decimal to a percent multiply by 100.
- To convert a percent to a decimal, divide by 100.
- Percentages are always related to the number 100.
- Decimals are written with a decimal point (.), percents are written with the percentage symbol (%), and ratios are written with a colon (:).
- A ratio is just like a fraction, decimal, or percent, in that it represents the parts of a whole.
- A ratio is a math statement of how two numbers compare.
- When reading a ratio, the colon is read as "is to."
- Proportions are used to write mathematical statements for two sets of numbers that are equal.
- When writing ratio proportions, we use a double colon (::) between two ratios.
- Ratios and proportions should be reduced to lowest terms.
- Cross multiplication is used to find unknown values in proportions.

# Chapter 7 Practice Test

**Answer *True* or *False* to the following statements:**

1. A percentage is a part of 100. _____

2. To convert a decimal to a percentage, you should always multiply by 50. _____

3. In order to express decimals as ratios, convert the decimal to a fraction. _____

4. Cross multiplication is used to find unknown values in proportions. _____

5. Ratios should never be reduced to lowest terms. _____

6. To express a ratio, always use the % symbol. _____

**Convert the following Decimals to Percents.**

1. 0.25 _____

2. 1 _____

3. 0.02 _____

4. 0.15 _____

5. 0.97 _____

**Convert the following Percents to Decimals.**

1. 401 _____

2. 1 _____

3. 45% _____

4. 225% _____

5. 6% _____

## Ratios

*Write the following as ratios.*

1. Your work 40 hours a week _____

2. $\dfrac{4}{9}$ _____

3. $2\dfrac{15}{17}$ _____

4. 0.15 _____

5. 82% _____

## Proportions

*Reduce the fraction or ratio to lowest terms; write your answers as proportions.*

1. $\dfrac{10}{500}$ _____

2. $7:49$ _____

3. $\dfrac{40}{360}$ _____

4. $2:4$ _____

5. $\dfrac{75}{300}$ _____

## Cross Multiplication

*Using cross multiplication, solve for the unknown value.*

1. $\dfrac{5}{7} = \dfrac{10}{?}$ _____

2. $\dfrac{?}{3} = \dfrac{4}{6}$ _____

3. $\dfrac{7}{9} = \dfrac{?}{54}$ _____

4. $\dfrac{?}{64} = \dfrac{1}{8}$ _____

5. $\dfrac{3}{5} = \dfrac{9}{?}$ _____

**Solve the Story Problem**

You are an LPN working weekends at an after-hours urgent care clinic. The clinic is open from 7:00 p.m. until 7:00 a.m. 7 days a week. Your work days are Sunday, Tuesday, Thursday, and Saturday, from 7:00 p.m. to 11:00 p.m.

The clinic saw 210 patients in the last 30 days; 120 were males and 90 were females. The clinic saw 45 male patients and 15 female patients between the ages of 18 and 25.

1. How many hours a week is the clinic open? —————

2. How many hours a week do you work? —————

3. Write a ratio of your hours to the clinic's open hours. —————

4. Using cross multiplication to solve for the unknown, then write you answer in a percent and round to a whole number. (That will be the percent of the clinic's open hour you work.) —————

5. What is the ratio of male patients to female patients; reduce your answer if possible? —————

6. Write a ratio proportion using your answers from question 5. —————

7. Using your reduced answer from question 5, write the ratio as a fraction, convert your fraction to a decimal, and then convert the decimal to a percent.

   Fraction —————

   Decimal —————

   Percent —————

# 8 Systems of Measurement

## INTRODUCTION

Different systems of measurement use specific unit types, each with their own names and value. The standard *household* system of measurement is the system commonly used in the United States. We are familiar with this system in our daily living. The *metric system* is used in the medical profession. As a nurse or allied health professional, you will need to know how to convert from one system of measurement to another. In chapter 8 you will learn different systems of measurement and how to convert between them, including working with temperatures and time.

## KEY TERMS

1. **Centi**  A prefix used in the metric system to represent one hundredth.
2. **Conversion**  A change from one system to another with the same or equal value.
3. **Gram**  A term used in the metric system to measure mass.
4. **Household System**  The system of measurement used in the United States.
5. **Kilo**  A prefix used in the metric system to represent one thousand.
6. **Liter**  A metric term used to describe volume.
7. **Metric System**  A system of measurement based on multiples of ten used in the medical industry and most countries outside the United States.
8. **Micro**  A prefix used in the metric system to represent one millionth.
9. **Milli**  A prefix used in the metric system to represent one thousandth.
10. **Unit of Measurement**  A division of any quantity that represents an accepted standard of measurement.

## WORKING WITH CONVERSIONS

As a nurse or allied health professional, you will work with conversions as a part of your daily responsibilities. Conversions are changing from one unit of measurement to another of equivalent value. An example would be making change for a $20 bill. Whether you make change using two $10 bills or using four $5.00 bills, you still have $20.00. You have converted from one type of bill to another. The key to working with conversions is to understand the value of the units you are converting from and converting to. We will cover conversions throughout this chapter as we learn the different systems of measurement.

# STANDARD HOUSEHOLD SYSTEM OF MEASUREMENT

The standard household system of measurement is the system commonly used in the United States for measuring and weighing items. In your home examples include a cup of milk, a gallon of milk or a quart of motor oil. A unit of measurement is a particular measurement or value, such as a teaspoon, tablespoon, ounce, cup, or pound. It can be notated by using a specific abbreviation. It is extremely important that you include the unit of measurement or correct abbreviation used to measure items when recording measurements. Now let's learn the standard household system of measurement for liquids using Table 8-1.

**TABLE 8-1  Standard Household System of Measurement**

| Unit of Measurement Liquids | Abbreviation | Equivalent Measures |
|---|---|---|
| drop | drop | |
| teaspoon | tsp. | 60 drops = 1 tsp. |
| tablespoon | tbsp. | 3 tsp. = 1 tbsp. |
| ounce | oz. | 2 tbsp. = 1 oz. |
| cup | cup, c | 8 oz. = 1 c. |
| pint | pt. | 2 c. = 1 pt. |
| quart | qt. | 2 pt. = 1 qt. |
| gallon | gal. | 4 qt. = 1 gal. |

Now that we know the standard household system of measurement for liquids, we can learn how to convert between different units of measurement. In order to perform conversions, we need to know the conversion factor. A conversion factor is the units that are being converting to and from. So, if we need to convert cups to ounces, our **conversion factor would be 8 ounces in 1 cup**. We can set up and solve our conversions using either fraction proportions or ratio proportions. Recall that we worked with proportions in Chapter 7.

Let's try one using each method, and then you can decide which method works best for you.

---

### EXAMPLE

**Using Fraction Proportion:** Convert 2 cups to ounces.

**STEP 1** Determine the conversion factor, and write it as a fraction. ALWAYS place the number **1** as your numerator and write it to the left of your equation. So, here our numerator is **1** cup, and our denominator is 8 ounces.

$$\frac{1 \text{ cup}}{8 \text{ ounces}} = —$$

**STEP 2** Set up your second fraction with the unknown value as the denominator and place it on the right side of the equation.

$$\frac{1 \text{ cup}}{8 \text{ ounces}} = \frac{2 \text{ cups}}{?}$$

**STEP 3** Cancel like units.

$$\frac{1 \text{ cup}}{8 \text{ ounces}} = \frac{2 \text{ cups}}{?}$$

**STEP 4** Cross multiply.

$$\frac{1}{8 \text{ ounces}} \diagup \frac{2}{?}$$

$1 \times ? = ?$

$8 \text{ ounces} \times 2 = 16 \text{ ounces}$

**STEP 5** Solve for the unknown.

$1 \times ? = ?$
8 ounces $\times$ 2 = 16 ounces
? = 16 ounces
Answer: 2 cups = 16 ounces

## EXAMPLE

**Using Ratio Proportion:** Convert 2 cups to ounces.

**STEP 1** Determine the conversion factor, **with 1 always to the left side of the first ratio**, and write the ratio to the left of your double colon in your equation.

<u>1 cup : 8 ounces</u> ::

**STEP 2** Set up the second ratio with the unknown to the right side of the second ratio, and write the ratio to the right of the double colon.

1 cup : 8 ounces :: <u>2 cups : ? ounces</u>

**STEP 3** Cancel like units.

1 cup : 8 ounces :: 2 cups : ?

**STEP 4** Multiply the outside values and inside values. (This is the same as if we cross multiplied using the fraction proportion method $\frac{1}{8 \text{ ounces}} \bowtie \frac{2}{?}$)

Inside values

1 : 8 ounces :: 2 : ?

Outside values
Outside values: $1 \times ? = ?$
Inside values: 8 ounces $\times$ 2 = 16 ounces

**STEP 5** Solve for the unknown.

Outside values: $1 \times ? = ?$
Inside values: 8 ounces $\times$ 2 = 16 ounces
? = 16 ounces
Answer: there are 16 ounces in 2 cups

Now let's try one more using each method.

## EXAMPLE

**Using Fraction Proportion:** Convert 2 cups to tablespoons.

First we need to determine how many tablespoons are in 1 cup. We know there are 2 tablespoons in 1 ounce, and that there are 8 ounces in 1 cup.

**STEP 1** Determine the conversion factor, and write it as a fraction. ALWAYS place the number 1 as your numerator and write it to the left of your equation.

$$\frac{1 \text{ ounce}}{2 \text{ tablespoons}} = —$$

**STEP 2** Set up your second fraction with the unknown value as the denominator, and place it on the right side of the equation.

$$\frac{1 \text{ ounce}}{2 \text{ tablespoons}} = \frac{8 \text{ ounces}}{?}$$

—*Continued next page*

*Continued—*

**STEP 3**  Cancel like units.

$$\frac{1 \text{ ounce}}{2 \text{ tablespoons}} = \frac{8 \text{ ounces}}{?}$$

**STEP 4**  Cross multiply.

$$\frac{1}{2 \text{ tablespoons}} \bowtie \frac{8}{?}$$

1 × ? = ?
8 tablespoons × 2 = 16 tablespoons

**STEP 5**  Solve for the unknown.

1 × ? = ?
8 tablespoons × 2 = 16 tablespoons
? = 16 tablespoons
Answer: 1 cup = 16 tablespoons

**STEP 6**  Solve the equation.

2 cups = ? tablespoons

We need to know how many tablespoons are in 2 cups. We know there are 16 tablespoons in 1 cup, so we can multiply our answer to our unknown in step 5 by 2.

*16 tablespoons* × 2 = 32 *tablespoons*

OR

We can set up another conversion factor equation and work steps 1 through 5 again.

Step 1 ⟶ $\dfrac{1 \text{ cup}}{16 \text{ tablespoons}}$ = $\dfrac{2 \text{ cups}}{?}$ ⟵ Step 2

Step 3 ⟶ $\dfrac{1 \text{ cup}}{16 \text{ tablespoons}}$ = $\dfrac{2 \text{ cups}}{?}$

Step 4 ⟶ $\dfrac{1}{16 \text{ tablespoons}} \bowtie \dfrac{2}{?}$

Step 5 ⟶ 1 × ? = ?
⟶ 16 tablespoons × 2 = 32 tablespoons

? = 32 tablespoons

Answer: 2 cups = 32 tablespoons

---

**E X A M P L E**

**Using Ratio Proportion:** Convert 2 cups to tablespoons.

First we need to determine how many tablespoons are in 1 cup. We know there are 2 tablespoons in one ounce, and 8 ounces in 1 cup.

**STEP 1**  Determine your conversion factor and write it to the left of your double colon in your equation.

1 ounce : 2 tablespoons ::

**STEP 2**  Set up your second ratio with the unknown to the right side of the second ratio, and write the ratio to the right of the double colon.

1 ounce : 2 tablespoons :: 8 ounces : ?

**STEP 3** Cancel like units.

1 ~~ounce~~ : 2 tablespoons :: 8 ~~ounces~~ : ?

**STEP 4** Multiply the outside values and inside values. (This is the same as if we cross multiplied using the fraction proportion method $\frac{1}{2\ tbsps.} \bowtie \frac{8}{?}$)

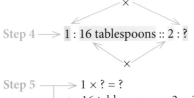

Inside values

1 : 2 tablespoons :: 8 : ?

Outside values

Outside values: $1 \times ? = ?$
Inside values: 2 tablespoons $\times$ 8 = 16 tablespoons

**STEP 5** Solve for the unknown.

Outside values: $1 \times ? = ?$
Inside values: 2 tablespoons $\times$ 8 = 16 tablespoons
? = 16 tablespoons
Answer: 1 cup = 16 tablespoons

**STEP 6** Solve the equation.

2 cups = ? tablespoons

We need to know how many tablespoons are in 2 cups. There are 16 tablespoons in 1 cup, so we can simply multiply our answer to our unknown in step 5 by 2.

16 tablespoons $\times$ 2 = 32 tablespoons

OR

We can set up another conversion factor equation. And work steps 1 through 5 again.

Step 1 ⟶ 1 cup : 16 tablespoons :: 2 cups : ? ⟵ Step 2

Step 3 ⟶ 1 cup : 16 tablespoons :: 2 cups : ?

Step 4 ⟶ 1 : 16 tablespoons :: 2 : ?

Step 5 ⟶ $1 \times ? = ?$
16 tablespoons $\times$ 2 = 32 tablespoons
? = 32 tablespoons
Answer: 2 cups = 32 tablespoons

## Practice Exercise 8-1   Answer the following questions about standard household measurements. Convert when needed and be sure to include the units with your answer (i.e., oz., tsp., c.).

1. How many ounces are in 1 cup?            _____

2. How many pints are in 2 quarts?          _____

3. How many teaspoons are in a tablespoon?  _____

4. How many drops are in 3 teaspoons?       _____

5. How many tablespoons are in 4 ounces?    _____

6. How many teaspoons are in 1 ounce?       _____

7. How many quarts are in one gallon?       _____

8. How many ounces are in 5 cups?           _____

**9.** How many cups are in 1 quart? _____

**10.** How many pints are in 3 quarts? _____

# METRIC SYSTEM OF MEASUREMENT

The metric system is used in all medical and scientific professions and is the system of measurement used in most countries. As previously stated, as a nurse or allied health professional, you will need to be able to convert between systems. The metric system is set up in multiples of 10, just like the number system used in the United States. This is called the customary system. The main difference is the terms used to identify values. When working with weights (solids), the metric system uses the term gram and the customary system uses the term pound. When working with volume (liquids) the metric system uses the term liter, and the customary system uses quart.

The metric system uses prefixes to identify values associated with grams and liters. Table 8-2 lists the metric system prefixes, terms, abbreviations, and values that are most commonly used in conversions needed to be performed by medical and allied health professionals.

**TABLE 8-2  Metric System Values**

| Prefix/Term | kilo- | gram | milli- | micro- |
|---|---|---|---|---|
| Abbreviations | kg | **g** | mg | mcg |
| Values | 1 kilogram (kg) = 1000 grams | **1 gram** | 1 gram = 1000 milligrams (mg) | 1 milligram = 1000 micrograms (mcg) |
| Prefix/Term | kilo- | **liter** | milli- | micro- |
| Abbreviations | kL | **L** | mL | mcL |
| Values | 1 kiloliter (kL) = 1000 liters | **1 liter** | 1 liter = 1000 milliliters (mL) | 1 milliliter = 1000 microliters (mcL) |

Looking at Table 8-2, we can see that each of the places on the scale has a value of 1000. If we need to convert within the metric system, we know that we are working in place values of 1000. When working with the metric system, you will **always** write your answers in decimal format.

When converting within the metric system, you can use a memory tool for converting grams and liters by writing the lines below:

For grams, write out:   kg   g   mg   mcg

Or,

For liters, write out:   kL   L   mL   mcL

Now if you need to convert from kilograms (kg) to milligrams (mg) or from microliters (mcL) to milliliters (mL), you can count how many place values you move to determine how many times you need to multiply or divide by 1000.

---

**EXAMPLE**

Convert from kilograms to milligrams:   kg   g   mg   mcg

Here we will move 2 place values to the right on our line. When we move to the right, we multiply. To convert from kilograms to milligrams, we need to multiply by 1000 two times (which is actually multiplying by 1,000,000).

---

**EXAMPLE**

Convert from microliters to milliliters:   kL   L   mL   mcL

Here we will move 1 place value to the left. When we move to the left, we divide. We need to divide by 1000.

Let's try converting within the metric system.

---

**EXAMPLE**

Convert 0.025 grams to milligrams

**STEP 1** Write out your line for grams:

  kg  g  mg  mcg

**STEP 2** Determine how many place values you need to move and in which directions.

  kg  g $\longrightarrow$ **mg**  mcg

You need to move 1 value place to the right, so you need to multiply by 1000.

**STEP 3** Perform your conversion by multiplying 0.025 g by 1000.

  0.025 g × 1000 = 25 mg

Let's do one more!

Convert 175 milliliters to liters

**STEP 1** Write out your line for liters:

  kL  L  mL  mcL

**STEP 2** Determine how many place values you need to move and in which directions.

  kL  **L** $\longleftarrow$ mL  mcL

You need to move 1 value place to the left, so you need to divide by 1000.

**STEP 3** Perform your conversion by dividing 175 mL by 1000.

  175 mL ÷ 1000 = 0.175 L

---

**Practice Exercise 8-2**  Convert the following within the Metric System.

1. Convert 0.025 mcg to mg        _____

2. Convert 0.0375 mL to L         _____

3. Convert 500 kg to g            _____

4. Convert 2500 g to mg           _____

5. Convert 750 mL to mcL          _____

6. Convert 0.005 mg to kg         _____

7. Convert 650 kL to L            _____

8. Convert 450 kg to g            _____

9. Convert 0.001 mL to L          _____

10. Convert 100 g to mg           _____

## CONVERTING BETWEEN STANDARD HOUSEHOLD AND METRIC SYSTEMS OF MEASUREMENTS

Now that we have learned how to convert **within** the household and metric systems, we can learn how to convert **between** the two systems. In order to correctly convert between the household and metric systems we need to learn the conversion factors of equivalent measures between the two systems listed in Table 8-3.

**TABLE 8-3  Household System and Metric System Equivalent Measures**

| Standard Household System | Metric System |
|---|---|
| **Unit of Measurement** | **Metric Equivalent Measures** |
| **Liquids** | |
| **drop** | **20 drops = 1 mL** |
| **teaspoon**<br>60 drops = 1 tsp. | **5 mL = 1 teaspoon** |
| **tablespoon**<br>3 tsp. = 1 tbsp. | **15 mL = 1 tablespoon** |
| **ounce**<br>2 tbsp. = 1 oz. | **30 mL = 1 ounce** |
| **cup**<br>8 oz. = 1 c. | **240 mL = 1 cup** |
| **Solids** | |
| **pound** | **1 kg = 2.2 pounds** |
| **1 teaspoon** | **5 grams** |
| **1 ounce** | **28.35 grams** |

Using Table 8-3, let's try converting between the standard household and metric systems.

---

**EXAMPLE**

Convert 2 teaspoons to mL

Looking at Table 8-3, we know there are 5 mL in 1 teaspoon. To determine how many mL are in 2 teaspoons, we multiply 5 mL by 2.

1 tsp. = 5 mL
5 mL × 2 = 10 mL

---

We can also solve our conversion using the fraction proportion or ratio proportion method.

## Fraction Proportion Method

Set up a conversion factor equation, and work following the 5 steps.

$$\text{Step 1} \longrightarrow \boxed{\frac{1\ \text{tsp}}{5\ \text{mL}} = \frac{2\ \text{tsp}}{?}} \longleftarrow \text{Step 2}$$

$$\text{Step 3} \longrightarrow \frac{1\ \text{tsp}}{5\ \text{mL}} = \frac{2\ \text{tsp}}{?}$$

$$\text{Step 4} \longrightarrow \frac{1}{5\ \text{mL}} \boxtimes \frac{2}{?}$$

$$\text{Step 5} \longrightarrow \begin{array}{l} 1 \times ? = ? \\ 5\ \text{mL} \times 2 = 10\ \text{mL} \\ ? = 10\ \text{mL} \end{array}$$

Answer: 2 teaspoons = 10 mL

## Ratio Proportion Method

Set up a conversion ratio proportion, and work the following 5 steps.

Step 1 ⟶ 1 tsp. : 5 mL :: 2 tsp. : ? ⟵ Step 2

Step 3 ⟶ 1 tsp : 5 mL :: 2 tsp : ?

$$\times$$

Step 4 ⟶ 1 : 5 mL :: 2 : ?

$$\times$$

Step 5 ⟶ 1 × ? = ?

5 mL × 2 = 10 mL

? = 10 mL

Answer: 2 teaspoons = 10 mL

Let's do another one more, to make sure we perfect it!

### EXAMPLE

Convert 4 ounces to mL

Looking at Table 8-3, we know there are 30 mL in 1 ounce. To determine how many mL are in 4 ounces, we multiply 30 mL by 4.

1 oz. = 30 mL
30 mL × 4 = 120 mL

We can also solve our conversion using the fraction proportion or ratio proportion method.

## Fraction Proportion Method

Set up a conversion factor equation and work the following 5 steps.

Step 1 ⟶ $\dfrac{1 \text{ oz.}}{30 \text{ mL}}$ = $\dfrac{4 \text{ oz.}}{?}$ ⟵ Step 2

Step 3 ⟶ $\dfrac{1 \text{ oz.}}{30 \text{ mL}} = \dfrac{2 \text{ oz.}}{?}$

Step 4 ⟶ $\dfrac{1}{30 \text{ mL}} \bowtie \dfrac{4}{?}$

Step 5 ⟶ 1 × ? = ?

30 mL × 4 = 120 mL

? = 120 mL

Answer: 4 ounces = 120 mL

## Ratio Proportion Method

Set up a conversion ratio proportion, and work the following 5 steps.

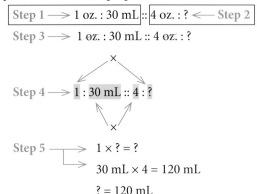

Answer: 4 ounces = 120 mL

**Practice Exercise 8-3**  Convert between the standard household and metric systems.

1. Convert 1 cup to mL                    _____

2. Convert 2 tbsp. to mL                  _____

3. Convert 15 mL to tsp.                  _____

4. Convert 360 mL to oz.                  _____

5. Convert 12 lbs. to kg                  _____

6. Convert 480 mL to cups                 _____

7. Convert 45 mL to tbsp.                 _____

8. Convert 6 tsp. to mL and grams         _____

9. Convert 5 oz. to mL and grams          _____

10. Convert 25 kg to lbs.                 _____

# TEMPERATURE

In the United States, we measure temperature in Fahrenheit (°F) and the metric system measures temperature in Celsius (°C). Again we need to know how to convert between the two systems. To convert temperatures, we use formulas. The formulas used to convert form Fahrenheit (°F) to Celsius (°C) and from Celsius (°C) to Fahrenheit (°F) are listed in Table 8-4.

**TABLE 8-4  Temperature Conversion Formulas**

| Fahrenheit (°F) to Celsius (°C) |
| :---: |
| °F − 32 ÷ 1.8 = °C |
| Celsius (°C) to Fahrenheit (°F) |
| °C × 1.8 + 32 = °F |

To convert temperature between systems, write out the formulas with answer blanks. Separate the steps to ensure you don't miss a step.

**EXAMPLE**

Convert 98.6 °F to °C

**STEP 1** Set up your formula with answer blanks:

°F − 32 ÷ 1.8 = °C
Becomes
_____ °F − 32 = _____, and then, _____ ÷ 1.8 = _____ °C

**STEP 2** Fill in the blanks and work the math!

98.6 °F − 32 = 66.6 and, 66.6 ÷ 1.8 = 37°C

Now let's convert from Celsius (°C) to Fahrenheit (°F).

**EXAMPLE**

Convert 40 °C to °F

**STEP 1** Set up your formula with answer blanks:

°C × 1.8 + 32 = °F

Becomes

_____ °C × 1.8 = _____, and then, _____ + 32 = _____ °F

**STEP 2** Fill in the blanks and work the math!

27.5 °C × 1.8 = 49.5, and then, 49.5 + 32 = 81.5 °F

**Practice Exercise 8-4**  Convert the temperatures (round to the nearest tenths when needed).

1. Convert 83.7 °F to °C          _____
2. Convert 17.8 °C to °F          _____
3. Convert 72.4 °F to °C          _____
4. Convert 38.5 °C to °F          _____
5. Convert 212 °F to °C           _____
6. Convert 98.6 °F to °C          _____
7. Convert 42.6 °C to °F          _____
8. Convert 125 °F to °C           _____
9. Convert 72.5 °C to °F          _____
10. Convert 63 °F to °C           _____

## TIME

The United States routinely uses a 12-hour clock time system. It is divided into 2 time periods. Each period is 12 hours. The time from midnight to noon is "a.m." and uses the numbers 1–11:59 followed by an "a.m." The time from noon to midnight is "p.m." using the numbers 1–11:59 "p.m." This differentiates between the two 12-hour time periods in a 24-hour day. Medical facilities use the 24-hour-clock time system. This is also referred to as military or universal time. The 24-hour-clock system is based on the 24-hour day. When working with the 24-hour-clock system, all times are recorded using 4 digits followed by the word "hours." For example, 9:15 a.m. is recorded as 0915 and read as "zero nine fifteen hours" in the 24-hour-clock system. Likewise, 10:00 a.m. is 1000 and read as "ten hundred hours" in the 24-hour-clock system. When using the 24-hour-clock system, the numbers are consecutive. It begins at 0100 and ends in 2400 with the first 12 hours 0100 through 1200, and after 12 noon 1300 through 2400. To determine the 24-hour clock system after 12 noon, add 1200 to the time. For example, 2:00 p.m. is recorded as 1400 hours in the 24-hour-clock system and read as "fourteen hundred hours." Subsequently, 2:30 p.m. is 1430 hours and read as "fourteen thirty hours." Table 8-5 lists the 12-hour-clock and 24-hour-clock systems.

**TABLE 8-5  12-Hour and 24-Hour Clock Systems**

| 12-Hour-Clock System | 24-Hour-Clock System |
| --- | --- |
| 1:00 a.m. | 0100 hours |
| 2:00 a.m. | 0200 hours |
| 3:00 a.m. | 0300 hours |
| 4:00 a.m. | 0400 hours |
| 5:00 a.m. | 0500 hours |
| 6:00 a.m. | 0600 hours |
| 7:00 a.m. | 0700 hours |
| 8:00 a.m. | 0800 hours |
| 9:00 a.m. | 0900 hours |
| 10:00 a.m. | 1000 hours |
| 11:00 a.m. | 1100 hours |
| 12:00 noon | 1200 hours |
| 1:00 p.m. | 1300 hours |
| 2:00 p.m. | 1400 hours |
| 3:00 p.m. | 1500 hours |
| 4:00 p.m. | 1600 hours |
| 5:00 p.m. | 1700 hours |
| 6:00 p.m. | 1800 hours |
| 7:00 p.m. | 1900 hours |
| 8:00 p.m. | 2000 hours |
| 9:00 p.m. | 2100 hours |
| 10:00 p.m. | 2200 hours |
| 11:00 p.m. | 2300 hours |
| 12:00 midnight | 2400 hours |

Let's try a few!

**EXAMPLES**

In the 12-hour-clock system, 11:17 a.m. converts to 1117 hours in the 24-hour-clock system, and is read as "eleven seventeen hours."

In the 12-hour-clock system, 3:45 p.m. converts to 1545 hours in the 24-hour-clock system, which is read as "fifteen forty five hours."

In the 12-hour-clock system, 7:00 p.m. converts to 1900 hours in the 24-hour-clock system and is read as "nineteen hundred hours."

**Practice Exercise 8-5**  Convert the following 12-hour-clock time to 24-hour-clock time.

1. 4:12 a.m.  _____

2. 5:19 p.m.  _____

3. 2:13 p.m.  _____

4. 7:32 a.m.  _____

5. 4:30 p.m.  _____

6. 1:56 a.m.  _____

7. 11:10 p.m.  _____

8. 6:40 p.m.  _____

9. 10:15 a.m.  _____

10. 9:30 p.m.  _____

## MANUAL MATH CORNER

### *The Corner of Mind and Math!*

When converting within the metric system, each place on the value scale has the value of 1000.

Look at the number 1000, how many zeros are there? 1000—Three, right!

To convert between metric system value places manually, you can simply move your decimal point 3 places.

**kg    g    mg    mcg**

For example, if you are converting from kilograms to grams we are moving to the right on the place value scale. You would move your decimal point 3 value places to the right!

Convert 0.3572 kilograms to grams

0.3572 kg = 357.2 g. We move the decimal 3 value places to the right!

## Recipes for success......

### SCENARIO 1

Your school is hosting a goodbye dinner for all the international exchange students before they return home to their native countries. All the dishes represent traditional cooking in different regions of the United States. Your class is making Jambalaya.

### Jambalaya with Sausage and Shrimp

*Convert the following ingredients to the metric system. Round your answer to the nearest tenths place.*

8 oz. hot or mild sausage  _____

1½ c. diced green pepper  _____

1½ c. diced red or yellow pepper  _____

1 lb. large peeled and divined shrimp  _____

2 tsp. salt  _____

3 tbsp. butter  _____

2½ tbsp. paprika  _____

1 tbsp. cayenne pepper  _____

1 bay leaf  _____

1 c. diced tomatoes  _____

2 c. diced green onions   _____

$1\frac{2}{3}$ c. uncooked brown rice   _____

3 c. chicken or vegetable stock   _____

## SCENARIO 2

Your dinner is a great success! All the students want the recipes to take back to their prospective countries. Everyone provides their recipes in Fahrenheit, but the international students ask for oven and refrigerator temperatures in Celsius.

*Convert the following temperatures from Fahrenheit to Celsius (round to the nearest tenths place when needed).*

**1.** Convert 350 °F   _____
**6.** Convert 72 °F   _____

**2.** Convert 425 °F   _____
**7.** Convert 32 °F   _____

**3.** Convert 42 °F   _____
**8.** Convert 275 °F   _____

**4.** Convert 450 °F   _____
**9.** Convert 325 °F   _____

**5.** Convert 500 °F   _____
**10.** Convert 400 °F   _____

---

**Nursing and Numbers**

Often body weights of patients are converted from pounds to kilograms.

Medicines are dosed many times by body weight. The pharmaceutical companies use kilograms because they manufacture for many countries and use the most commonly used system worldwide. We learned that system is metric. The nurse will need to know how to convert from the customary system to the metric system.

A pharmaceutical example is: "give 5 mg/kg" of a drug. This is read as "give 5 mg for each kilogram of body weight."

When obtaining and recording patient temperatures, Celsius is often used and you will need to be able to quickly convert from Fahrenheit to Celsius.

---

# CHAPTER SUMMARY

- The United States uses the standard household system of measurement.
- Most other countries and the medical and scientific community use the metric unit of measurement system.
- The metric system uses multiples of 10.
- The metric system uses prefixes to denote different values.
- Nurses and allied health professionals need to be able to convert between the metric and standard household systems of measurement.
- Conversion equations can be solved using the fraction proportion or ratio proportion method.
- Celsius and Fahrenheit are both used to measure temperature.
- The formula for converting Fahrenheit to Celsius is °F − 32 ÷ 1.8 = °C.
- The formula for converting Celsius to Fahrenheit is °C × 1.8 + 32 = °F.
- Most medical facilities use the 24-hour-clock time system, which can be referred to as military or universal time.
- The 24-hour-clock time system is based on the 24-hour day.

# Chapter 8 Practice Test

**Answer *True* or *False* to the following statements:**

1. One tablespoon is equal to 10 milliliters.                          _____

2. The medical community uses the metric system of measurement.    _____

3. The 24-hour-clock time system can be called military time.         _____

4. Four quarts are equivalent to 1 pint.                              _____

5. Most countries outside the United States use the standard
   household system of measurement.                                  _____

6. The metric system uses prefixes to denote different values.        _____

## Household

1. How many pints are in 4 quarts?                                    _____

2. How many teaspoons are in 2 tablespoons?                          _____

3. How many drops are in 1 teaspoon?                                  _____

4. How many ounces are in 3 cups?                                     _____

5. How many teaspoons are in 5 ounces?                               _____

## Metric

1. Convert 0.0075 mcg to mg      _____

2. Convert 0.750 mL to L         _____

3. Convert 500 g to mg           _____

4. Convert 3.75 g to mg          _____

5. Convert 0.0025 L to mL        _____

*Convert between the standard household and metric systems.*

1. Convert 1 cup to mL      _____

2. Convert 2 tbsp. to mL    _____

3. Convert 15 mL to tsp.    _____

4. Convert 360 mL to oz.    _____

5. Convert 12 lbs. to kg    _____

## Temperature

*Convert the temperatures (round to the nearest tenths when needed).*

1. Convert 78.3 °F to °C    _____

2. Convert 18.2 °C to °F    _____

3. Convert 94.6 °F to °C    _____

4. Convert 25.8 °C to °F    _____

5. Convert 100 °F to °C     _____

## Time

*Convert the following 12-hour-clock time to 24-hour-clock time.*

**1.** 5:30 a.m. _____

**2.** 8:50 p.m. _____

**3.** 11:49 p.m. _____

**4.** 3:15 a.m. _____

**5.** 7:45 p.m. _____

### Solve the Story Problem

You are working as a patient care technician in an inpatient physical rehabilitation center. A new patient is transferred to your facility for 2 weeks of therapy to strengthen his left leg. He is 4 days postoperation following a total knee replacement. The patient is 67 years old, 5 foot 8 inches tall, and weighs 75 kg. The patient needs round-the-clock care to help reduce the risk of infection to the surgical site, maintain pain management, and reduce swelling of the left leg. The admission orders are as follows:

Take vital signs at 0600 hours, 1200 hours, 1800 hours, and 2400 hours. If temperature is greater than 38.3 °C, administer 0.375 grams of acetaminophen. If temperature is greater than 39.4 °C, contact the physician on call for the orthopedic surgeon group at 1-555-4DR-BONE.

Administer 1 gram of intravenous antibiotics over the period of 1 hour at 0800 hours and 2000 hours.

Administer 800 mg of oral anti-inflammatory medication at 0700 hours, 1500 hours, and 1900 hours.

Administer 2 mg of pain medication at 0400 hours, 1000 hours, 1600 hours, and 2200 hours.

**1.** Convert the times to take the patient's vital signs to the 12-hour-clock time system _____

**2.** Convert the temperatures to Fahrenheit _____

**3.** Convert the patient's weight to pounds _____

**4.** Convert 1 gram of antibiotics to milligrams _____

# 9 Putting It All Together

## INTRODUCTION

The basic math skills presented in the previous eight chapters have given you a solid base of basic math skills to build from as you advance your mathematical skill sets. This may include various calculation methods and formulas used in your career as a nurse or allied health professional. Chapter 9 is a comprehensive review of all the skills we covered in Chapters 1 through 8. Congratulations on mastering over 30 basic math skills! Great Job!

## UNDERSTANDING NUMBERS, STORY PROBLEMS, AND NUMBERING SYSTEMS

Reading for numbers, and understanding story problems and numbering systems, is a very important skill. Nurses and allied health professionals need these skills in every aspect of their career. In Chapter 1, we learned Arabic and Roman Numbering systems, number values, and how to identify and extract pertinent information from story problems.

**Practice Exercise 9-1**  Complete the following exercises based on Chapter 1.

1. List the eight steps needed to solve a story problem.

   1. _____     5. _____

   2. _____     6. _____

   3. _____     7. _____

   4. _____     8. _____

2. List the number of digits in each number.

   765 _____     52 _____     90432 _____

3. Fill in the missing numbers in the counting line.

   4's: 4, ___, 12, 16, 20, ___, ___, 32, ___, 40.

4. Express the Arabic digits 6 and 7 as a fraction _____

5. List the rules for Roman Numerals.

   1. _____

   2. _____

   3. _____

Convert the following Roman Numerals to Arabic Numbers.

**6.** X _____          **8.** XCV _____

**7.** LXXXI _____      **9.** XVIII _____

Convert the following Arabic numbers to Roman Numerals.

**10.** 77 _____         **12.** 45 _____

**11.** 500 _____

# BASIC OPERATIONS AND WHOLE NUMBERS

In Chapter 1, we learned how numbering systems worked. In Chapter 2, we learned how those systems can be used in the basic mathematical operations of addition, subtraction, multiplication, and division. We realized that nurses and allied health professionals use these systems every day. We also learned how to check our work for accuracy.

**Practice Exercise 9-2**  Complete the following exercises based on Chapters 1 and 2.

**1.** $18 + 8 =$ _____     **3.** $2 \times 54 =$ _____

**2.** $43 - 31 =$ _____    **4.** $264 \div 12 =$ _____

Fill in the blanks.

**5.** Use _____ to double-check a division quotient.

**6.** Subtraction is the opposite of _____.

**7.** $X \times XIV =$ _____

**8.** $C - XXII =$ _____

Four people split the driving and cost of a 236-mile trip. Gas for the trip cost $144.00.

**9.** How many miles does each person drive? _____

**10.** If two drivers each drive 42 miles, how many miles are left to get to their destination? _____

# FRACTIONS AND MIXED NUMBERS

In Chapters 1 and 2 we learned about number values and how to do equations with whole numbers. The basic multiplication and division skills learned in Chapter 2 assisted us in Chapter 3 to understand parts of whole numbers.

**Practice Exercise 9-3**  Complete the following exercises based on Chapters 1 to 3.

**1.** Express the following digits as a whole number 8, 5, 7 _____

**2.** Express the following digits as an improper fraction 9, 7 _____

**3.** Convert the fraction from your answer in question 2 to a mixed number _____

Fill in the blanks.

**4.** A _____ is the term used to describe the top number in a fraction.

**5.** A whole number and fraction expressed together is known as a _____.

6. _____ and _____ are important concepts used when working with fractions.

7. Reduce the fraction to lowest terms.

   1. $\dfrac{88}{99} =$                      2. $\dfrac{15}{25} =$

8. Convert the following mixed number to an improper fraction.

   1. $8\dfrac{4}{15}$ _____                    2. $3\dfrac{5}{6}$ _____

9. Write the following fraction in Roman Numerals $\dfrac{5}{47}$ _____

10. List the three types of fractions.

   1. _____        2. _____        3. _____

# BASIC OPERATIONS WITH FRACTIONS

In Chapter 4, we use our basic operations skills learned in previous chapters to understand fractions.

**Practice Exercise 9-4**   Complete the following exercises based on Chapters 1 to 4.

1. $45 \times 97$ _____

2. Convert the following to a mixed number.

   $\dfrac{80}{45}$ _____

3. Reduce the following fraction to lowest terms.

   $\dfrac{42}{63}$ _____

4. $873 - 21$ _____

5. $\dfrac{7}{9} + \dfrac{13}{18}$ _____

6. $\dfrac{\text{III}}{\text{X}} \div \dfrac{\text{I}}{\text{V}}$ _____

7. Find the lowest common denominator for the following sets of fractions.

   1. $2\dfrac{1}{4}$ and $\dfrac{4}{5}$ _____          2. $\dfrac{1}{6}$ and $\dfrac{8}{9}$ _____

8. $\dfrac{1}{6} \times \dfrac{12}{15}$ _____

**Fill in the blanks.**

9. To _____ a fraction is to turn it upside down.

10. A _____ denominator is needed to solve addition or subtraction equations with fractions.

# WORKING WITH DECIMALS

In Chapter 5, we learned that decimals, like fractions, are parts of a whole. We also learned the place values, how to convert between decimals and fractions, and the rules for rounding. Now we can put these skills together with the skills we learned in Chapters 1 through 4.

**Practice Exercise 9-5**   Complete the following exercises based on Chapters 1 to 5.

Identify the place value for the bold and underlined numbers.

1. 92**8**3.645 _____          3. 5**6**01.782 _____

2. 1092.83**4** _____

Solve the following fraction and mixed number equations. Convert your answers to Arabic numbers when needed. Convert that answer to a decimal and round to the nearest tenth.

4. $\dfrac{XII}{XX} - \dfrac{V}{XX}$ _____          5. $1\dfrac{5}{6} + 2\dfrac{1}{3}$ _____

Work the following fraction equations and reduce to lowest terms. Convert your answer to a decimal and round to the nearest hundredth.

6. $\dfrac{5}{15} \times \dfrac{2}{6}$ _____          7. $\dfrac{15}{75} \div \dfrac{1}{3}$ _____

Convert the following decimals to fractions; reduce to lowest terms. Convert your answers to Roman numerals.

8. 7.75 _____          10. 4.05 _____

9. 2.5 _____

## BASIC OPERATIONS WITH DECIMALS

In Chapter 6 we learned how important working with decimals is to the daily practice of a nurse or allied health professional. Placing the decimal point in the incorrect value place can lead to a serious or even deadly patient consequence. As a nurse or allied health professional, you must master accuracy when working with multiple equation types to ensure patient safety.

**Practice Exercise 9-6**   Solve the following decimal equations. Show your answers rounded to the nearest hundredths and nearest tenths.

1.    25.75          3.    167.543          5.    450.225
    +42.8                + 94.035              −375.05

2.    1859.10          4.    2301.006
    −  682.07            −1032.6

Solve the following decimal equations and round to the nearest hundredth. Convert your answers to an **improper fraction**, a proper fraction, or mixed number. Remember to reduce your answers to lowest terms.

6. $3.750 \div 1.45 =$ _____

7. $1.225 \times 1.5 =$ _____

8. $45.50 \div 2.25 =$ _____

9. $542.71 \times 1.2 =$ _____

10. $6.45 \div 2.5 =$ _____

## PERCENTS, RATIOS, AND PROPORTIONS

In Chapter 7, we learned that percents and ratios are like decimals and fractions, in that they represent a portion of a whole. We learned that proportions are statements showing two ratios are equal. Lastly, we learned that cross multiplication is used to find unknown values in proportions. Now we can incorporate everything we learned in Chapter 7 with what we learned in Chapters 1 through 6.

**Practice Exercise 9-7** Solve the following equations, using all the basic mathematical skills you learned in Chapters 1 through 7.

Convert the decimals to percents.

  **1.** 4.75 _____                   **2.** 0.87 _____

Convert the percents to decimals and then fractions. Reduce to lowest terms when needed.

  **3.** 397% _____              **4.** 175% _____

Write the following as ratios. Convert to fractions and reduce to lowest terms. Write your final answers as ratio proportions.

  **5.** 80 is to 100 _____         **6.** 15 is to 45 _____

Reduce the fraction and write your answers as fraction proportions.

  **7.** $\dfrac{5}{15}$ _____             **8.** $\dfrac{6}{48}$ _____

Use cross multiplication to solve for the unknown.

  **9.** $\dfrac{8}{12} = \dfrac{?}{3}$ _____       **10.** $\dfrac{?}{81} = \dfrac{2}{9}$ _____

# SYSTEMS OF MEASUREMENT

In Chapter 8, we learned the different systems of measurement, units of measurement abbreviations, and how to convert within and between systems, including temperatures and time. Everything we learned in Chapter 8, combined with Chapters 1 through 7, has given you a solid building block of basic math skills required of a nurse or allied health professional.

**Practice Exercise 9-8** Solve the following using the method of your choice.

  **1.** How many tablespoons are in 3 ounces? _____

  **2.** Convert 115 pounds to kilograms (round to the nearest tenths). _____

  **3.** How many drops are in 10 mL? _____

  **4.** How many mL are in XII ounces? _____

  **5.** Convert 7500 milliliters to liters. _____

  **6.** Convert 0.25 grams to milligram. _____

  **7.** Convert 9:45 a.m. to 24-hour-clock time. _____

  **8.** Convert 1745 hours to 12-hour-clock time. _____

**Fill in the Blanks**

  **9.** Write the formula used to convert from °F to °C. _____

**10.** Write the formula used to convert from °C to °F. _____

---

**Nursing and Numbers**

Every career starts on day one. Everyone has a first day. You are starting your career as a nurse. The math you have learned from this book is your foundation from which you will build on every day. Practice your math skills until they are second nature. As you practice and study math, you will take great satisfaction in solving problems.

# COMPREHENSIVE EXAM (CHAPTERS 1 TO 8)

1. A denominator is the top number in a fraction.

2. A Roman numeral letter can only repeat itself four times.

3. When rounding, if the number to the right of the desired place value is 1 through 4, do not change the value of the number.

4. Place value is not an important concept in math.

5. A nurse or allied health professional should be able to convert between different systems of measurement.

6. There are six basic types of fractions.

7. The sum of two or more numbers can be described as the total.

8. A liter is a term used in the standard household measurement system.

9. Roman numerals use letters to represent number values.

10. Most medical facilities use the military or universal time system.


*Fill in the blanks.*

11. There are _____ steps to solving a story problem.

12. A _____ is a digit that has no place value, always a zero.

13. Any number written to the _____ of the decimal point represents a whole number.

14. A _____ is a whole number and fraction expressed together.

15. The medical community uses the _____ as the unit of measurement.

16. The Arabic number system consists of _____ digits.

17. _____ ounces is equal to one cup.

18. 2:00 PM is expressed as _____ in military time.

19. One tablespoon is equal to _____ milliliters.

20. To determine a fractional decimal value, _____ your numerator by your denominator.


*Match the correct math term to its definition.*

| | | |
|---|---|---|
| 21. | Gram | Any amount that is a part of 100 |
| 22. | Quotient | The value of a number in multiples of 10, based on the digit's placement |
| 23. | Dividend | A change from one system to another with the same or equal value |
| 24. | Standard household System | A metric term used to describe volume |
| 25. | Total | The sum of two or more numbers |
| 26. | Proportion | A mathematical term to describe the number "*that is being divided*" |
| 27. | Place value | A mathematical term to describe the answer to a division equation |
| 28. | Percent | A mathematical term referring to two equal fractions or ratios |
| 29. | Liter | The system of measurement used in the United States |
| 30. | Conversion | A term used in the metric system to measure mass |

*Solve the following equations. Reduce to lowest terms, change to mixed numbers. Answer Roman in Roman numerals and Arabic numbers. Give decimal answers to the tenth place.*

**31.** $81 - 35.6 =$

**32.** $99.756 \times \dfrac{3}{5} =$

**33.** $\dfrac{9}{10} + \dfrac{1}{12} + \dfrac{2}{5} =$

**34.** $\dfrac{10}{47} \div \dfrac{6}{13} = \dfrac{130}{282} =$

**35.** $845 \div 114 =$

**36.** $67°C =$

**37.** $10 \ tsp =$

**38.** $10 \ tbls =$

**39.** $78.67 + 51.56 + 9.23 =$

**40.** $8\dfrac{3}{10} \times 1\dfrac{3}{4} =$

**41.** $\dfrac{49}{77} =$

**42.** $231 \times 15 =$

**43.** $7{:}00 \ \text{PM} =$

**44.** $\dfrac{3}{10} = \dfrac{15}{?}$

**45.** $35 \ g =$

**46.** $87°F =$

**47.** $\text{LXV} - \text{XXXIV} =$

**48.** $305.228 + 213.4 + 0.006 =$

**49.** $199 \div 23 =$

**50.** $\dfrac{11}{15} - 0.06 =$

**51.** $\dfrac{\text{XVII}}{\text{L}} + \dfrac{\text{III}}{\text{X}} = \dfrac{\text{XVI}}{\text{XXV}} =$

**52.** $4\dfrac{2}{5} + 7\dfrac{13}{15} =$

**53.** $513 + 23 =$

**54.** $\dfrac{5}{7} \times \dfrac{11}{12} \times 0.951 =$

**55.** $256.214 \times 132.46 =$

**56.** $23000 \ mL =$

**57.** $142 \ pounds =$

**58.** $12 - \dfrac{9}{32} =$

**59.** $2300 \ hours =$

**60.** $8 \times 67 =$

**61.** $0.33 =$

**62.** $\text{DXX.IX} \div \text{LXIII.V} =$

**63.** $108 \ kg =$

## Solve the Story Problem

You are working at the local health department as a licensed practical nurse in the patient education and disease prevention department. There has been a recent nationwide increase in the number of child cases of whooping cough (pertussis). Your supervisor is informed by the State Board of Health that the Centers for Disease Control and Prevention (CDC) is conducting a study on the number of children in your community who have not been immunized against the disease and the reasons why, if known.

You are asked to compare the state's records of vital statistics to determine how many children live in your community and compare that list to the state's immunization records. Once you have a master list of the children living in your community who have not been immunized, you are asked to contact the parents and determine why the children have not been immunized against pertussis. Your report must be turned in to your supervisor in 2 weeks.

Your report shows there are 372 children between the ages of 2 and 4 years of age, and that 103 have not been immunized. Over the course of the study, you were able to contact the parents of 96 of the children. You prepare the report of your findings with the reasons why these children have not received the pertussis vaccine. The report shows that 71 did not receive vaccines because of lack of means (no insurance and lack of income), 3 did not believe in vaccines, they felt they would cause more harm than good, and 2 indicated that immunizations were not given because of religious beliefs. The remaining parents indicated they were unaware that their children needed to have immunizations until they started school at the age of 5.

Based on your report, the state will determine if your community is eligible for a grant that would help fund an immunization clinic to provide the pertussis vaccine to children in your community. To receive the grant, your community must have 85% or more of the unimmunized children categorized as uninsured, underinsured, or unaware.

If your community is eligible for the grant, it will be receive enough vaccine to immunize the 103 unimmunized children in your community. The community will also receive $25.00 per unimmunized child to offset the cost of staffing and administration costs. Each immunization contains 0.5 mL of the vaccine and there are 5 mL of vaccine per vial.

**64.** Write a ratio of the number of children living in your community and the number of children who have not received the pertussis vaccine. _____

**65.** Write a fraction for the number of children not immunized because of lack of means as your numerator, and the total number of children not immunized as your denominator. Determine the conversion factor needed to set up an equation to solve for the unknown percentage of unimmunized children who did not get immunized because of the lack of means. Solve the equation (round to the nearest hundredth). _____

**66.** Determine the percent of unimmunized children who were not vaccinated because the parents were unaware of the need before age 5 (round to the nearest hundredths). _____

**67.** Write a fraction for the number of children not immunized because of lack of means, and a fraction for the number of children not immunized because of parents being unaware of the age requirements for vaccines. Use the total number of unimmunized children as the denominator for both fractions. Add the two fractions and then determine the percentage of children unimmunized based on the sum of the two fractions (round to the nearest hundredths). _____

**68.** Based on your report, is your community eligible for a grant to fund an immunization clinic? _____

**69.** How many immunizations can be given from each vial of vaccine? _____

**70.** What is the total amount of grant money your health department will receive? _____

# Answer Key

## Chapter 1: Understanding Numbers, Story Problems, and Numbering Systems

### Practice Exercise 1-1

1. One case, 1 case

    Seventy-five dollar, Seventy-five dollars and zero cents

2. Ten boxes

    1 full case, a case, one case, 1 case

3. Fifty gloves

    A box, one box, 1 box

### Practice Exercise 1-2

1. One case, $75.00

    10, boxes of gloves

    Each thin cardboard box, 50

2. Purple

    Latex-free

    Thin cardboard

### Practice Exercise 1-3

**STEP 1** How much would one of each glove cost?

**STEP 2** You are reading a medical supply company sales ad, and they have a case of purple latex-free gloves on sale for $75.00 a case. You need to determine if the sale price is a good value for your office. Each case contains 10 thin cardboard boxes of gloves. Each box of gloves costs $7.50, and each box contains 50 purple latex-free gloves.

**STEP 3** Divide cost of box by number of gloves.

**STEP 4** Each case of gloves costs $75.00.

   Each case contains 10 thin cardboard boxes of gloves.

**STEP 5** Each box of gloves costs 7.50.

   Each box contains 50 gloves.

**STEP 6** 7.50/50 = ?

**STEP 7** 7.50/50 = 0.15

**STEP 8** Each glove would cost 0.15 cents.

## Practice Exercise 1-4

1. Combine the digits 6, 14, 20 to create the new number of 61420

   Add the numbers 6 + 14 + 20 = 40

2. Combine the digits 15, 30, 45 to create the new number of 153035

   Add the numbers 15 + 30 + 45 = 90

## Practice Exercise 1-5

| | | |
|---|---|---|
| 1. XX | 3. CC | 5. DXXX |
| 2. III | 4. XXIII | |

## Practice Exercise 1-6

| | | |
|---|---|---|
| 1. 9 | 3. 99 | 5. 4 |
| 2. 900 | 4. 44 | |

## Practice Exercise 1-7

| | | |
|---|---|---|
| 1. CM | 3. XLIX | 5. XCIX |
| 2. XL | 4. XXIV | |

## Practice Exercise 1-8

| | | |
|---|---|---|
| 1. 35 | 3. 55 | 5. 62 |
| 2. 18 | 4. 520 | |

## Practice Exercise 1-9

| | | |
|---|---|---|
| 1. 17 | 3. 707 | 5. 42 |
| 2. 80 | 4. 39 | |

## Review Exercises

| | | |
|---|---|---|
| 1. 40 | 5. 97 | 9. 32 |
| 2. 79 | 6. 35 | 10. 56 |
| 3. 501 | 7. 81 | |
| 4. 44 | 8. 900 | |

Convert the following Arabic Numbers into Roman Numerals.

| | | |
|---|---|---|
| 1. LXXX | 5. XXIV | 9. XXXVIII |
| 2. DCCCXC | 6. LI | 10. M |
| 3. VII | 7. XLIV | |
| 4. LXXVI | 8. XX | |

## Recipes for success......

| **SCENARIO 1** | **SCENARIO 2** |
| --- | --- |
| **Ingredients** | **Ingredients** |
| 15, 14 and ½ | IV |
| 2 and ½ | II and ss |
| 1–2 | X and ss |
| 10 | II and ss, (VIII) |
| ½, 1 | III |
| 2 and ½ | III |
| 2 and ½ | II and ss, (II) |
| 1 and ½ | I and ss |
| 1 and ½ | I and ss |
| ½ | |

**SCENARIO 2**

1 and 2

2 and ½

5

3 and ½

10, (6 oz.)

5, (15 oz.)

**SCENARIO 3**

**1.** 1 cup

**2.** 9 cups

**STEP 1** *Read:*  1.  How much bleach will you need?

2.  How much water will you need?

**STEP 2** *Read Scenario:* You are a laboratory assistant and your supervisor has asked you to make a recipe card to use for making 1 part bleach to 9 part water cleaning solution for the laboratory counter tops and blood drawing tables. You need to make 10 cups of solution total. You have two gallons of distilled water and a half gallon of bleach in the lab to use to make your solution. To write the recipe for the bleach and water solution, you need to determine how much water and how much bleach will you need, and how much bleach will be needed from each gallon.

**STEP 3** To write the recipe for the bleach and water solution you need to determine how much water and how much bleach will you need. We need 10 cups of solution made up of 9 parts of water and 1 part bleach. 10 cups = 10 parts.

**STEP 4** You have two gallons of distilled water and a half gallon of bleach in the lab to use to make your solution.

**STEP 5** To make 10 cups of 1 part bleach to 9 parts water solution, pour _____ cup/s water into a large spill-proof container, then slowly add _____ cup/s of bleach, secure cap tightly, and mix carefully.

**STEP 6** 10 cups – 9 cups = ? cups

**STEP 7** 10 cups of solution – 9 parts water = 1 part bleach, each part is equal to 1 cup

**STEP 8** 1.  How much bleach will you need?    1 cup

2.  How much water will you need?    9 cups

## Chapter 1 Practice Test

Twenty seven years old

Three months

One hundred and seventy-three pounds

Ninety-eight point four degrees

Twenty-five dollars

**STEP 1** Read the questions

**STEP 2** Read the story

**STEP 3** Interpret what is being asked

**STEP 4** Identify extraneous information

**STEP 5** Identify and extract information needed to set up the equation

**STEP 6** Set up the equation

**STEP 7** Solve the equation

**STEP 8** Solve the story problem

**Solve the Story Problems**

**STEP 1** *Read:* What time would you need to leave your home next Friday in order to drive 2 hours to the convention center from your home?

**STEP 2** *Read story:* You are scheduled to attend a continuing education conference next weekend. The conference is out of town, and it will take you 2 hours to drive to the convention center from your home. You are expected to attend a dinner reception at 6:00 p.m. on Friday night at the convention center. You want to arrive early to check into your room and freshen up before the dinner reception so you plan to arrive at 4:30 p.m.

**STEP 3** Determine what time you need to leave in order to arrive at 4:30.

**STEP 4** next Friday, 6:00 p.m.

**STEP 5** 2 hours to drive to the convention center from your home, arrive at the convention center at 4:30 p.m.

**STEP 6** 4:30 p.m. – 2 hours = ? p.m.

**STEP 7** 4:30 – 2 hours = 2:30 p.m.

**STEP 8** You need to leave no later than 2:30 p.m.

**List the number of digits in each number:**

| | | |
|---|---|---|
| **1.** 2 | **3.** 3 | **5.** 4 |
| **2.** 3 | **4.** 5 | **6.** 3 |

**Fill in the missing numbers in the counting lines:**

| | | |
|---|---|---|
| **1.** 8, 16, 22 | **4.** 10, 25, 40, | **7.** 3/5 |
| **2.** 81622 | **5.** 102540 | **8.** 0.14 |
| **3.** 8, 16, 22, 46 | **6.** 10, 25, 40, 75 | |

Answer *True* or *False* to the following statements:

| | | |
|---|---|---|
| **1.** T | **4.** F | **7.** T |
| **2.** F | **5.** T | **8.** F |
| **3.** T | **6.** F | |

Convert the following Arabic numbers to Roman Numerals.

| | | |
|---|---|---|
| **1.** XXXIII | **5.** CI | **9.** LXXIII |
| **2.** LXXXII | **6.** DCCI | **10.** XC |
| **3.** V | **7.** LIV | |
| **4.** XIX | **8.** LXVI | |

Convert the following Roman Numerals to Arabic numbers.

| | | |
|---|---|---|
| **1.** 49 | **5.** 93 | **9.** 16 |
| **2.** 530 | **6.** 550 | **10.** 1500 |
| **3.** 15 | **7.** 51 | |
| **4.** 50 | **8.** 3 | |

# Chapter 2:  Basic Operations and Whole Numbers

## Practice Exercise 2-1

| | | |
|---|---|---|
| **1.** 28 | **3.** 8 | **5.** 7 |
| **2.** 14 | **4.** 15 | |

## Practice Exercise 2-2

**1.**
```
  456
  420
+ 003
  879
```

**2.**
```
  365
+ 132
  497
```

**3.**
```
  602
  313
+ 074
  989
```

**4.**
```
  703
  020
+ 005
  728
```

**5.**
```
  123
+ 325
  448
```

## Practice Exercise 2-3

**1.**
```
  4531
  2551
+ 0091
  7173
```

**2.**
```
  002
+ 999
 1001
```

**3.**
```
  4871
+ 6711
 11582
```

**4.**
```
  194
+ 067
  261
```

**5.**
```
  981
  755
+ 046
 1782
```

## Practice Exercise 2-4

1.  450
    +082
    532

2.  960
    +489
    1449

3.  1556
    +0123
    1679

4.  565
    +214
    779

5.  678
    043
    +089
    810

6.  9829
    +1433
    11262

7.  811
    056
    +009
    876

8.  333
    087
    045
    +012
    477

9.  165
    123
    076
    +040
    404

10. 862
    113
    +067
    1042

## Practice Exercise 2-5

1.  84
    −41
    43

2.  66
    −13
    53

3.  56
    −22
    34

4.  92
    −81
    11

5.  49
    −17
    32

## Practice Exercise 2-6

1.  547
    −269
    278

2.  898
    −499
    399

3.  765
    −88
    677

4.  1857
    −949
    908

5.  375
    −368
    7

## Practice Exercise 2-7

1.  67
    −56
    11

2.  961
    −288
    673

3.  657
    −259
    398

4.  69
    −23
    46

5.  4152
    −653
    3499

6.  148
    −52
    96

7.  784
    −365
    419

8.  6212
    −1989
    4223

9.  3571
    −755
    2816

10. 5840
    −2237
    3603

## Practice Exercise 2-8

| | × 1 | | × 2 | | × 3 |
|---|---|---|---|---|---|
| 1 | 1 | 1 | 2 | 1 | 3 |
| 2 | 2 | 2 | 4 | 2 | 6 |
| 3 | 3 | 3 | 6 | 3 | 9 |
| 4 | 4 | 4 | 8 | 4 | 12 |
| 5 | 5 | 5 | 10 | 5 | 15 |
| 6 | 6 | 6 | 12 | 6 | 18 |
| 7 | 7 | 7 | 14 | 7 | 21 |
| 8 | 8 | 8 | 16 | 8 | 24 |
| 9 | 9 | 9 | 18 | 9 | 27 |

| | × 4 | | × 5 | | × 6 |
|---|---|---|---|---|---|
| 1 | 4 | 1 | 5 | 1 | 6 |
| 2 | 8 | 2 | 10 | 2 | 12 |
| 3 | 12 | 3 | 15 | 3 | 18 |
| 4 | 16 | 4 | 20 | 4 | 24 |
| 5 | 20 | 5 | 25 | 5 | 30 |
| 6 | 24 | 6 | 30 | 6 | 36 |
| 7 | 28 | 7 | 35 | 7 | 42 |
| 8 | 32 | 8 | 40 | 8 | 48 |
| 9 | 36 | 9 | 45 | 9 | 54 |

| | × 7 | | × 8 | | × 9 |
|---|---|---|---|---|---|
| 1 | 7 | 1 | 8 | 1 | 9 |
| 2 | 14 | 2 | 16 | 2 | 18 |
| 3 | 21 | 3 | 24 | 3 | 27 |
| 4 | 28 | 4 | 32 | 4 | 36 |
| 5 | 35 | 5 | 40 | 5 | 45 |
| 6 | 42 | 6 | 48 | 6 | 54 |
| 7 | 49 | 7 | 56 | 7 | 63 |
| 8 | 56 | 8 | 64 | 8 | 72 |
| 9 | 63 | 9 | 72 | 9 | 81 |

## Practice Exercise 2-9

**1.** Repeat the value of 1 four times.

Multiplication: $1 \times 4 = 4$

Addition: $1 + 1 + 1 + 1 = 4$

Counting: 1, 2, 3, 4

**2.** Repeat the value of 2 three times.

Multiplication: $2 \times 3 = 6$

Addition: $2 + 2 + 2 = 6$

Counting: 2, 4, 6

**3.** Repeat the value of 3 five times.

Multiplication: $3 \times 5 = 15$

Addition: $5 + 5 + 5 = 15$

Counting: 3, 6, 9, 12, 15

**4.** Repeat the value of 4 two times.

Multiplication: $4 \times 2 = 8$

Addition: $4 + 4 = 8$

Counting: 4, 8

5. Repeat the value of 5 seven times.

   Multiplication: $5 \times 7 = 35$

   Addition: $5 + 5 + 5 + 5 + 5 + 5 + 5 = 35$

   Counting: 5, 10, 15, 20, 25, 30, 35

6. Repeat the value of 6 six times.

   Multiplication: $6 \times 6 = 36$

   Addition: $6 + 6 + 6 + 6 + 6 + 6 = 36$

   Counting: 6, 12, 18, 24, 30, 36

7. Repeat the value of 7 three times.

   Multiplication: $7 \times 3 = 21$

   Addition: $7 + 7 + 7 = 21$

   Counting: 7, 14, 21

8. Repeat the value of 8 five times.

   Multiplication: $8 \times 5 = 40$

   Addition: $8 + 8 + 8 + 8 + 8 = 40$

   Counting: 8, 16, 24, 32, 40

9. Repeat the value of 9 four times.

   Multiplication: $9 \times 4 = 36$

   Addition: $9 + 9 + 9 + 9 = 36$

   Counting: 9, 18, 27, 36

## Practice Exercise 2-10

$$
\begin{array}{r}
1. \quad 2 \\
\times 5 \\
\hline 10
\end{array}
$$

$$
\begin{array}{r}
2. \quad 7 \\
\times 9 \\
\hline 63
\end{array}
$$

$$
\begin{array}{r}
3. \quad 10 \\
\times 4 \\
\hline 40
\end{array}
$$

$$
\begin{array}{r}
4. \quad 15 \\
\times 5 \\
\hline 75
\end{array}
$$

$$
\begin{array}{r}
5. \quad 12 \\
\times 7 \\
\hline 84
\end{array}
$$

$$
\begin{array}{r}
6. \quad 25 \\
\times 10 \\
\hline 00 \\
+ 250 \\
\hline 250
\end{array}
$$

$$
\begin{array}{r}
7. \quad 100 \\
\times 50 \\
\hline 000 \\
+ 5000 \\
\hline 5000
\end{array}
$$

$$
\begin{array}{r}
8. \quad 47 \\
\times 20 \\
\hline 00 \\
+ 940 \\
\hline 940
\end{array}
$$

$$
\begin{array}{r}
9. \quad 250 \\
\times 3 \\
\hline 750
\end{array}
$$

$$
\begin{array}{r}
10. \quad 60 \\
\times 3 \\
\hline 180
\end{array}
$$

## Practice Exercise 2-11

1. $75 \div 15 =$

   Answer: 5, $5 \times 15 = 75$

2. $842 \div 4 =$

   Answer: 210 r 2, $210 \times 4 = 840$, $840 + 2 = 842$

3. $37 \div 3 =$

   Answer: 12 r 1, $12 \times 3 = 36$, $36 + 1 = 37$

4. $250 \div 50 =$

   Answer: 5, $5 \times 50 = 250$

5. $56 \div 8 =$

   Answer: 7, $7 \times 8 = 56$

**6.** $749 \div 100 =$

Answer: 7 r 49, $7 \times 100 = 700$, $700 + 49 = 749$

**7.** $144 \div 12 =$

Answer: 12, $12 \times 12 = 144$

**8.** $480 \div 30 =$

Answer: 16, $16 \times 30 = 480$

**9.** $81 \div 9 =$

Answer: 9, $9 \times 9 = 81$

**10.** $17 \div 4 =$

Answer: 4 r 1, $4 \times 4 = 16$, $16 + 1 = 17$

## Recipes for success......

### SCENARIO 1

**Ingredients**

| | |
|---|---|
| 3 cups flour | 9 cups |
| 1½ cups sugar | 4½ cups |
| 1 egg | 3 eggs |
| 1 cup vegetable shortening | 3 cups |
| 1 teaspoon salt | 3 teaspoons |
| 1 pinch of cinnamon | 3 pinches |
| 3 teaspoons cornstarch | 9 teaspoons |
| 1 teaspoon baking powder | 3 teaspoons |
| 4 cups of blackberries | 12 cups |

### SCENARIO 2

How much does each employee owe for the bill?    $12.00

## Chapter 2 Practice Test

**Answer *True* or *False* to the following statements:**

| | | |
|---|---|---|
| **1.** F | **5.** T | **9.** F |
| **2.** F | **6.** F | **10.** T |
| **3.** T | **7.** T | |
| **4.** T | **8.** F | |

**Solve the following equations. Line them up in columns and show your work next to them. Double check your answers using a calculator.**

1.  $\begin{array}{r} 88 \\ +65 \\ \hline 153 \end{array}$

2.  $\begin{array}{r} 943 \\ -637 \\ \hline 306 \end{array}$

3.  $\begin{array}{r} 47 \\ \times 29 \\ \hline 1363 \end{array}$

4.  $\begin{array}{r} 20 \\ \times\ 7 \\ \hline 140 \end{array}$

5.  $233 \div 6 = 38\ r\,5$

6.  $\begin{array}{r} 790 \\ \times\ 16 \\ \hline 12640 \end{array}$

7.  $\begin{array}{r} 253 \\ -\ 53 \\ \hline 200 \end{array}$

8.  $\begin{array}{r} 533 \\ -186 \\ \hline 347 \end{array}$

9.  $\begin{array}{r} 169 \\ +443 \\ \hline 612 \end{array}$

10. $\begin{array}{r} 562 \\ \times\ 13 \\ \hline 7306 \end{array}$

11. $\begin{array}{r} 2345 \\ +\ 123 \\ \hline 2468 \end{array}$

12. $\begin{array}{r} 84 \\ \times 21 \\ \hline 1764 \end{array}$

13. $\begin{array}{r} 569 \\ -279 \\ \hline 290 \end{array}$

14. $\begin{array}{r} 652 \\ -231 \\ \hline 421 \end{array}$

15. $\begin{array}{r} 712 \\ +745 \\ \hline 1457 \end{array}$

16. $\begin{array}{r} 200 \\ \times\ 76 \\ \hline 15200 \end{array}$

17. $\begin{array}{r} 214 \\ +\ 89 \\ \hline 303 \end{array}$

18. $\begin{array}{r} 1111 \\ \times\ 85 \\ \hline 94435 \end{array}$

19. $\begin{array}{r} 432 \\ -254 \\ \hline 178 \end{array}$

20. $\begin{array}{r} 417 \\ \times\ 96 \\ \hline 40032 \end{array}$

**Solve the following equations. Use multiplication to check your answer. Show your work next to each problem.**

1.  $843 \div 82 = 10\ r\,23$

2.  $984 \div 60 = 16\ r\,24$

3.  $854 \div 2 = 427$

4.  $199 \div 10 = 19\ r\,9$

5.  $655 \div 5 = 131$

6.  $754 \div 65 = 11\ r\,40$

7.  $240 \div 12 = 20$

8.  $989 \div 7 = 141\ r\,2$

**Using your skills from Chapter 1, solve the following equations. WRITE YOUR ANSWERS IN ROMAN NUMERALS.**

1.  XXIV + LVI = LXXX

2.  CM − XLV = DCCCLV

3.  XL × XIX = DCCLX

**Solve the Story Problem**

You are asked to conduct inventory on the medical supply room. Your supervisor gives you a list of the minimum number of each item that needs to be on hand at all times. You are to inform her if any items fall below the minimum number and by how many. You inventory the gloves first. The minimum number of boxes of small gloves is 6, medium gloves is 8, and large gloves is 10. In the supply room, you count 6 boxes of large gloves, 5 boxes of small gloves, and 9 boxes of medium gloves.

1.  Does the number of boxes of large gloves fall below the minimum number required to have on hand?   *Yes*

    If so, by how many boxes?   4

2.  Does the number of boxes of medium gloves fall below the minimum number required to have on hand?   *No*

    If so, by how many boxes?   0

3. Does the number of boxes of small gloves fall below the minimum number required to have on hand?     *Yes*

   If so, by how many boxes?     1

   What is the total number of boxes of gloves below the minimum number required?     *5*

# Chapter 3: Fractions and Mixed Numbers

## Practice Exercise 3-1

1. $\frac{1}{3}$

2. $\frac{5}{9}$

3. $\frac{7}{7}$

4. $\frac{13}{20}$

5. $\frac{5}{8}$

## Practice Exercise 3-2

1. $\frac{4}{3}$

2. $\frac{7}{5}$

3. $\frac{12}{6}$

4. $\frac{13}{8}$

5. $\frac{3}{2}$

## Practice Exercise 3-3

1. $1\frac{6}{12}, 1\frac{1}{2}$

2. $1\frac{4}{5}$

3. $3\frac{1}{2}$

4. 1

5. $3\frac{2}{7}$

## Practice Exercise 3-4

1. $\frac{23}{4}$

2. $\frac{43}{12}$

3. $\frac{20}{7}$

4. $\frac{31}{16}$

5. $\frac{28}{3}$

## Practice Exercise 3-5

1. $\frac{4}{5}$

2. $\frac{2}{3}$

3. $\frac{4}{5}$

4. $\frac{1}{9}$

5. $\frac{3}{8}$

## Recipes for success......

**SCENARIO 1**

1. 4

2. 8

3. $\frac{28}{32}$

4. $\frac{7}{8}$

5. 10

6. $\frac{5}{40}$

7. $\frac{1}{8}$

**SCENARIO 2**

1. $\frac{10}{20} = \frac{1}{2}$

2. $\frac{180}{9} = 20$ (20 is the number of servings per chili maker).

3. $\frac{715}{143} = 5$ ($5.00 is the donation price for each participant).

# Chapter 3 Practice Test

Answer *True* or *False* to the following statements:

1. T      3. F      5. T

2. F      4. F      6. T

Express the following as a Proper Fraction. Use the highlighted sections as the numerator. If applicable reduce to lowest terms.

1. $\frac{6}{12} = \frac{1}{2}$      3. $\frac{6}{22} = \frac{3}{11}$      5. $\frac{8}{18} = \frac{4}{9}$

2. $\frac{16}{20} = \frac{4}{5}$      4. $\frac{14}{21} = \frac{2}{3}$

Convert the following Improper Fractions to Mixed Numbers and reduce to the lowest terms.

1. $1\frac{39}{44}$      4. $3\frac{21}{25}$      7. $18\frac{3}{4}$

2. $2\frac{3}{16}$      5. $1\frac{1}{87}$      8. $1\frac{4}{5}$

3. $3\frac{7}{20}$      6. $11\frac{1}{13}$

Convert the following Mixed Numbers to Improper Fractions.

1. $\frac{38}{12}$      4. $\frac{25}{13}$      7. $\frac{42}{19}$

2. $\frac{12}{5}$      5. $\frac{41}{9}$      8. $\frac{17}{3}$

3. $\frac{62}{8}$      6. $\frac{14}{12}$

Reduce the following fractions to the lowest terms.

1. $\frac{1}{3}$      4. $\frac{5}{6}$      7. $\frac{1}{3}$

2. $\frac{7}{8}$      5. $\frac{2}{8} = \frac{1}{4}$      8. $\frac{1}{5}$

3. $\frac{1}{2}$      6. $\frac{1}{3}$

Solve the Story Problem

1. $\frac{4}{1}$

2. $\frac{3900}{150} = \$26.00$ (Each child will get 4 immunizations at $6.50, $6.50 × 4 = $26.00)

3. 110

4. $27\frac{5}{110} = 27\frac{1}{22}$ (110 immunizations ÷ 4 per child = 27.5 children immunized)

# Chapter 4: Basic Operations with Fractions

## Practice Exercise 4-1

1. $2\frac{1}{2}$

2. $1\frac{4}{25}$

3. $\frac{7}{10}$

4. $4\frac{1}{4}$

5. $\frac{8}{11}$

6. $\frac{1}{9}$

7. $\frac{8}{57}$

8. $\frac{12}{17}$

9. $\frac{18}{94} = \frac{9}{47}$

10. $\frac{8}{20} = \frac{2}{5}$

## Practice Exercise 4-2

1. $42, \frac{59}{42} = 1\frac{17}{42}$

2. $24, \frac{9}{24} = \frac{3}{8}$

3. $27, \frac{17}{27}$

4. $21, \frac{29}{21} = 1\frac{8}{21}$

5. $40, \frac{67}{40} = 1\frac{27}{40}$

## Practice Exercise 4-3

1. $1\frac{11}{18}$

2. $1\frac{12}{15} = 1\frac{4}{5}$

3. $1\frac{13}{16}$

4. $1\frac{17}{28}$

5. $1\frac{13}{16}$

6. $\frac{4}{33}$

7. $\frac{5}{54}$

8. $\frac{1}{18}$

9. $\frac{8}{6} = 1\frac{1}{3}$

10. $\frac{10}{32} = \frac{5}{16}$

## Practice Exercise 4-4

1. $3\frac{7}{20}$

2. $1\frac{41}{60}$

3. $1\frac{7}{22}$

4. $4\frac{7}{24}$

5. $3\frac{3}{26}$

6. $7\frac{8}{45}$

7. $\frac{3}{8}$

8. $6\frac{19}{48}$

9. $2\frac{10}{21}$

10. $2\frac{3}{104}$

## Practice Exercise 4-5

1. $\frac{35}{104}$

2. $\frac{29}{120}$

3. $\frac{198}{65} = 3\frac{3}{65}$

4. $\frac{28}{76} = \frac{7}{19}$

5. $\frac{1935}{104} = 18\frac{63}{104}$

6. $\frac{112}{153}$

7. $\frac{36}{169}$

### Practice Exercise 4-6

1. $\frac{27}{26} = 1\frac{11}{16}$     3. $\frac{65}{168}$     5. $\frac{49}{10} = 4\frac{9}{10}$

2. $\frac{180}{115} = 1\frac{65}{115} = 1\frac{13}{23}$     4. $\frac{88}{8} = 11$

## Recipes for success......

### SCENARIO 1

**Ingredients**

| | |
|---|---|
| $\frac{1}{2}$ cup of butter, melted | $\frac{3}{8}$ cups |
| $3\frac{1}{2}$ cups sugar | $2\frac{5}{8}$ cups |
| 3 eggs (beaten) | $2\frac{1}{4}$ eggs (2 eggs is practical for cooking purposes) |
| 1 can condensed tomato soup $\left(10\frac{1}{2}\text{ oz.}\right)$ (Please answer in ounces) | $7\frac{7}{8}$ oz. |
| $2\frac{1}{4}$ teaspoon cinnamon | $1\frac{11}{16}$ teaspoons |
| $2\frac{2}{3}$ teaspoons nutmeg | 2 teaspoons |
| 2 teaspoons baking soda | $1\frac{1}{2}$ teaspoons |
| 2 teaspoons salt | $1\frac{1}{2}$ teaspoons |
| 3 cups raisins | $2\frac{1}{4}$ cups |
| $2\frac{1}{2}$ cups chopped nuts | $1\frac{7}{8}$ cups |
| $4\frac{1}{2}$ cups flour | $3\frac{3}{8}$ cups |

### SCENARIO 2

| | |
|---|---|
| How much is left? | $243.36 |
| How much did you spend on books? | $81.12 |

## Chapter 4 Practice Test

Answer *True* or *False* to the following statements:

1. T     3. F     5. T

2. F     4. F     6. T

Solve the following fraction equations. Reduce your answer to Mixed numbers and/or lowest terms fractions.

1. $4\frac{32}{85}$

2. $11\frac{11}{15}$

3. $22\frac{16}{143}$

4. $3\frac{71}{114}$

5. $17\frac{8}{20} = 17\frac{2}{5}$

6. $1\frac{58}{72} = 1\frac{29}{36}$

7. $3\frac{34}{99}$

8. $4\frac{43}{70}$

9. $3\frac{9}{44}$

10. $3\frac{198}{230} = 3\frac{99}{115}$

11. $2\frac{34}{119}$

12. $4\frac{37}{168}$

13. $1\frac{219}{330}$

14. $8\frac{18}{35}$

15. $1\frac{147}{153} = 1\frac{49}{51}$

16. $3\frac{24}{220} = 3\frac{6}{55}$

17. $6\frac{12}{17}$

18. $7\frac{1}{19}$

19. $4\frac{13}{30}$

20. $9\frac{32}{153}$

Solve the Story Problem

1. $\frac{12}{15} + \frac{56}{60} + \frac{2}{30} = \frac{48}{60} + \frac{56}{60} + \frac{4}{60} = \frac{108}{60} \; 1\frac{48}{60} = 1\frac{4}{5}$

2. $\frac{108}{60} - \frac{2}{30} = \frac{108}{60} - \frac{4}{60} = \frac{104}{60} \; 1\frac{44}{60} = 1\frac{11}{15}$

# Chapter 5: Working with Decimals

## Practice Exercise 5-1

1. 4 is in the tens place

2. 9 is in the hundreds place

3. 5 is in the thousandths place

4. 1 is in the thousands place

5. 0 is in the tenths place

6. 2 is in the ones place

7. 4 is in the hundredths place

8. 9 is in the hundreds place

9. 3 is in the tenths place

10. 5 is in the thousands place

## Practice Exercise 5-2

1. 2.75

2. 0.25

3. 3.6

4. 0.2

5. 4.5

## Practice Exercise 5-3

1. $6\frac{75}{100}$

2. $\frac{5}{10} = \frac{1}{2}$

3. $\frac{25}{100} = \frac{1}{4}$

4. $1\frac{7}{10}$

5. $3\frac{3}{10}$

## Practice Exercise 5-4

1. 1.5

2. 0.2

3. 3.1

4. 0.141

5. 1.8

### Recipes for success......

| SCENARIO 1 | SCENARIO 2 |
|---|---|
| 2.25 | $83.33 |
| 1.5 | |
| 1.75 | |
| 0.67 or 0.7 | |
| 3.67 or 3.7 | |
| 2.33 or 2.3 | |
| 0.25 | |
| 0.83 or 0.8 | |

## Chapter 5 Practice Test

Answer *True* or *False* to the following statements:

| | | |
|---|---|---|
| **1.** T | **3.** F | **5.** T |
| **2.** F | **4.** T | **6.** F |

Identify the place value for the bold underlined numbers.

| | |
|---|---|
| **1.** 6 is in the ones place | **6.** 6 is in the tens place |
| **2.** 7 is in the hundredths place | **7.** 9 is in the hundreds place |
| **3.** 9 is in the hundreds place | **8.** 3 is in the thousandths place |
| **4.** 3 is in the tenths place | **9.** 1 is in the thousands place |
| **5.** 4 is in the thousands place | **10.** 3 is in the tenths place |

Convert the following Fractions to Decimals; round to the appropriate place value when needed.

| | | |
|---|---|---|
| **1.** 3.166 = 3.2 | **5.** 4.333 = 4.3 | **9.** 3.75 |
| **2.** 0.4 | **6.** 0.5 | **10.** 5.2 |
| **3.** 7.75 | **7.** 2.210 = 2.21 | |
| **4.** 1.923 = 2.0 | **8.** 5.666 = 5.7 | |

Convert the following Decimals to Fractions; reduce to lowest terms when needed.

| | | |
|---|---|---|
| **1.** $4\frac{25}{100} = 4\frac{1}{4}$ | **5.** $9\frac{5}{100} = 9\frac{1}{20}$ | **9.** $6\frac{4}{10} = 6\frac{2}{5}$ |
| **2.** $7\frac{5}{10} = 7\frac{1}{2}$ | **6.** $2\frac{5}{10} = 2\frac{1}{2}$ | **10.** $\frac{25}{1000} = \frac{1}{40}$ |
| **3.** $1\frac{20}{100} = 1\frac{1}{5}$ | **7.** $\frac{8}{10} = \frac{4}{5}$ | |
| **4.** $\frac{75}{100} = \frac{3}{4}$ | **8.** $1\frac{25}{100} = 1\frac{1}{4}$ | |

Solve the Story Problem

| | |
|---|---|
| **1.** 1/2, 0.5 | **3.** 2/3, 0.67 |
| **2.** 6/10, 0.6 | **4.** Sick waiting rooms 2/4, 0.5 |
| | Postprocedure waiting room 1/4, 0.25 |
| | Main waiting room 1/4, 0.25 |

# Chapter 6: Basic Operations with Decimals

## Practice Exercise 6-1

**1.**     255.09
         +  54.8
         309.89

**2.**     389.2
         −122.08
         267.12

**3.**     42.240
         +39.06
         81.30

**4.**   801.006
         −773.01
          27.996

**5.**     92.50
         −25.101
         67.399

**6.**   855.123
         +  66.94
         922.063

**7.**   186.742
         −  25.101
         161.641

**8.**     255.09
         +  54.8
         309.89

**9.**     389.32
         −122.08
         267.24

**10.**    42.240
         +39.06
         81.30

## Practice Exercise 6-2

**1.** 135.44

**2.** 38.37

**3.** 71.93

**4.** 110.53

**5.** 380.91

**6.** 5.88

**7.** 7.69

**8.** 6.41

**9.** 1.38

**10.** 7.25

## Recipes for success......

**SCENARIO 1**

**1.** Yes

**2.** $3.36

**3.** $50.34

**4.** $0.44 \times 15 = \$6.60$

**5.** $14.25

**6.** $0.03

**7.** $9.00

**8.** 10

**9.** $89.97

**SCENARIO 2**

**Ingredients**

| | |
|---|---|
| 4 cucumbers (sliced into 24 slices each) | 2 cucumbers |
| 8 oz. onion and chive-flavored cream cheese spread | 4 oz. cheese spread |
| ½ cup ranch salad dressing | ¼ c. ranch dressing |
| ¼ teaspoon garlic powder | ⅛ tsp. garlic powder |
| ¼ teaspoon fresh cracked black pepper | ⅛ tsp. black pepper |
| 1 teaspoon fresh chopped parsley | ½ tsp. parsley |
| 1 teaspoon fresh minced dill sprigs | ½ tsp. dill |
| 48 slices of multigrain bread | 24 slices of bread |
| Petite round cookie cutter | |

## Chapter 6 Practice Test

Answer *True* or *False* to the following statements:

**1.** F          **3.** T                    **5.** F

**2.** F          **4.** T

Add and Subtract.

**1.**     67.43
      +92.40
      159.83

**6.**   221.221
      − 99.999
      121.222

**2.**   271.05
      − 87.35
      183.70

**7.**     2.538
      +889.75
      892.288

**3.**     42.62
      +21.88
      64.50

**8.**     79.78
      −78.79
      .99

**4.**   199.36
      −  8.90
      190.46

**9.**   90.003
      + 8.61
      98.613

**5.** 592.637
      + 81.02
      673.657

**10.**    47.69
      −23.987
      23.703

Multiply and Divide (*round your answer to the nearest tenth*).

**1.** $95.2 \times 18.5 = 1761.2$          **6.** $764.32 \div 84.13 = 9.1$

**2.** $67.987 \div 4.222 = 16.1$          **7.** $.333 \times 71.21 = 23.7$

**3.** $152.3 \times .065 = 9.9$          **8.** $6.33 \div 1.964 = 3.2$

**4.** $84.90 \div 21.7 = 3.9$          **9.** $53.1 \times 2.621 = 139.2$

**5.** $456.1 \times .188 = 85.7$          **10.** $995.3 \div 2.75 = 361.9$

Solve the Story Problem

**1.** $50.00          **3.** $9.98          **5.** $20.92

**2.** $117.40          **4.** $11.50

# Chapter 7: Percents, Ratios, and Proportions

## Practice Exercise 7-1

**1.** 397%          **3.** 5%          **5.** 150%

**2.** 83%          **4.** 33%

## Practice Exercise 7-2

**1.** 0.75          **3.** 2.46          **5.** 0.03

**2.** 1.12          **4.** 0.25

## Practice Exercise 7-3

**1.** 8:24          **3.** 7:4          **5.** 75:100

**2.** 2:7          **4.** 50:100

## Practice Exercise 7-4

**1.** 75 : 100 :: 3 : 4          **3.** 15 : 45 :: 1 : 3          **5.** 8 : 24 :: 1 : 3

**2.** $\dfrac{50}{100} = \dfrac{1}{2}$          **4.** $\dfrac{12}{144} = \dfrac{1}{12}$

## Practice Exercise 7-5

**1.** ? = 5, $\dfrac{5}{25} = \dfrac{1}{5}$          **3.** ? = 3, $\dfrac{9}{12} = \dfrac{3}{4}$          **5.** ? = 21, $\dfrac{3}{7} = \dfrac{9}{21}$

**2.** ? = 18, $\dfrac{18}{36} = \dfrac{9}{18}$          **4.** ? = 15, $\dfrac{27}{45} = \dfrac{3}{5}$

## Recipes for success......

### SCENARIO 1

What is the total number of guests expected with the added 15%? (Round your answer).    58

You need 6.5 lbs. of flour to make all the pancakes. The flour only comes in 5-lb bags, so you need to buy two 5-lb bags, giving you a total of 10 lbs. of flour. What percentage of the flour will NOT be used?    35%

If the flour costs $3.47 per 5-lb bag and you are getting a 12% discount on each bag, what is the total cost of the flour?    $6.10

Turkey sausage links are $6.30 for a package containing 20. If each guest has three sausages, how many total packages do you need to purchase?    9

Write a ratio of total guests to total sausage.    58:174

What is the total price on the sausage you need to purchase?    $56.70

If you have a coupon for $1.00 off each package, what is the percentage off each package?    16% (1.008)

### SCENARIO 2

| | |
|---|---|
| 2 ½ cups flour | 2.5 cups |
| ½ cup sugar | 0.5 cup |
| ½ teaspoon baking soda | 0.5 teaspoon |
| ¼ teaspoon salt | 0.25 teaspoon |
| 2 eggs | 2.0 eggs |
| 1 cup walnuts | 1.0 cup |
| 2 bananas | 2.0 bananas |
| ⅔ cup butter | 0.67 cup |
| 1 cup powdered sugar | 1.0 cup |

## Chapter 7 Practice Test

Answer *True* or *False* to the following statements:

| | | |
|---|---|---|
| **1.** T | **3.** T | **5.** F |
| **2.** F | **4.** T | **6.** F |

Convert the following Decimals to Percents.

| | | |
|---|---|---|
| **1.** 25% | **3.** 2% | **5.** 97% |
| **2.** 100% | **4.** 15% | |

Convert the following Percents to Decimals.

| | | |
|---|---|---|
| **1.** 4.01 | **3.** 0.45 | **5.** 0.06 |
| **2.** 100% | **4.** 2.25 | |

Ratios

| | | |
|---|---|---|
| **1.** 40:168 | **3.** 49:17 | **5.** 82:100 |
| **2.** 4:9 | **4.** 152:1000 | |

Proportions

**1.** $\dfrac{10}{500} = \dfrac{1}{50}$   **3.** $\dfrac{40}{360} = \dfrac{1}{9}$   **5.** $\dfrac{75}{300} = \dfrac{1}{4}$

**2.** $7 : 49 :: 1 : 7$   **4.** $2 : 4 :: 1 : 2$

Cross Multiplication

**1.** $? = 14, \dfrac{5}{7} = \dfrac{10}{14}$   **3.** $? = 42, \dfrac{7}{9} = \dfrac{42}{54}$   **5.** $? = 15, \dfrac{3}{5} = \dfrac{9}{15}$

**2.** $? = 2, \dfrac{2}{3} = \dfrac{4}{6}$   **4.** $? = 8, \dfrac{8}{64} = \dfrac{1}{8}$

Solve the Story Problem

| | | |
|---|---|---|
| **1.** 84 | **4.** 19% | **7.** Fraction $\dfrac{3}{4}$ |
| **2.** 16 | **5.** 90 : 120, 3 : 4 | Decimal 0.75 |
| **3.** 16:84 | **6.** 90 : 120 :: 3 : 4 | Percent 75% |

# Chapter 8: Systems of Measurement

## Practice Exercise 8-1

| | |
|---|---|
| **1.** 8 oz. | **6.** 6 tsp. = 1 oz. |
| **2.** 4 pt. | **7.** 4 qt. = 1 gal. |
| **3.** 3 tsp. = 1 tbsp. | **8.** 40 oz. = 5 c. |
| **4.** 180 drops = 3 tsp. | **9.** 4 c. = 1 qt. |
| **5.** 8 tbsp. = 4 oz. | **10.** 6 pints = 3 quarts |

## Practice Exercise 8-2

1. 0.000025 mg
2. 0.0000375 L
3. 5000 g
4. 2500000 mg
5. 750000 mcL
6. 0.000000005 kg
7. 650000 L
8. 450000 g
9. 0.000001 L
10. 100000 mg

## Practice Exercise 8-3

1. 240 mL
2. 30 mL
3. 3 tsp.
4. 12 oz.
5. 5.45 lbs.
6. 2 cups
7. 3 tbsp.
8. 30 mL, 30 g
9. 150 mL, 141.75 g
10. 55 lbs.

## Practice Exercise 8-4

1. 28.7 °C
2. 64 °F
3. 22.4 °C
4. 101.3 °F
5. 100 °C
6. 37 °C
7. 108.68 °F, rounds to 108.7 °F
8. 51.666 °C, rounds to 51.7 °C
9. 162.5 °F
10. 17.2 °C

## Practice Exercise 8-5

1. 0412 hours
2. 1719 hours
3. 1413 hours
4. 0732 hours
5. 1630 hours
6. 0156 hours
7. 2310 hours
8. 1840 hours
9. 1015 hours
10. 2130 hours

## Recipes for success......

**SCENARIO 1**

**Ingredients**

| | |
|---|---|
| 8 oz. hot or mild sausage | 226.8g |
| 1½ c. diced green pepper | 340.2 g |
| 1 ½ c. diced red or yellow pepper | 340.2 g |
| 1 lb. large peeled and divined shrimp | 453.6 g, rounds 464 g |
| 2 tsp. salt | 10 g |
| 3 tbsp. butter | 45 g |
| 2 ½ tbsp. paprika | 37.5 g |
| 1 tbsp. cayenne pepper | 15 g |
| 1 bay leaf | 1 |
| 1 c. diced tomatoes | 226.8 g |
| 2 c. diced green onions | 453.6 g |
| 1 ⅔ c. uncooked brown rice | 376.5 g |
| 3 c. chicken or vegetable stock | 720 mL |

**SCENARIO 2**

| | | | |
|---|---|---|---|
| **1.** Convert 350 °F | 176.7 °C | **6.** Convert 72 °F | 22.2 °C |
| **2.** Convert 425 °F | 218.3 °C | **7.** Convert 32 °F | 0 °C |
| **3.** Convert 42 °F | 5.6 °C | **8.** Convert 275 °F | 135 °C |
| **4.** Convert 450 °F | 232.2 °C | **9.** Convert 325 °F | 162.8 °C |
| **5.** Convert 500 °F | 260 °C | **10.** Convert 400 °F | 204.4 °C |

# Chapter 8 Practice Test

Answer *True* or *False* to the following statements:

| | | |
|---|---|---|
| **1.** F | **3.** T | **5.** F |
| **2.** T | **4.** F | **6.** T |

Household

| | | |
|---|---|---|
| **1.** 8 pt. | **3.** 60 drops = 1 tsp. | **5.** 30 tsp. = 5 oz. |
| **2.** 6 tsp. = 2 tbsp. | **4.** 720 oz. = 3 c. | |

Metric

| | | |
|---|---|---|
| **1.** 7.5 mg | **3.** 0.5 mg | **5.** 2.5 mL |
| **2.** 750 L | **4.** 3750 mg | |

Convert between the household and metric systems

| | | |
|---|---|---|
| **1.** 240 mL | **3.** 3 tsp. | **5.** 5.45 lbs. |
| **2.** 30 mL | **4.** 12 oz. | |

Temperature

| | | |
|---|---|---|
| **1.** 25.7 °C | **3.** 34.7 °C | **5.** 37.7 °C |
| **2.** 64.8 °F | **4.** 78.4 °F | |

Time

| | | |
|---|---|---|
| **1.** 0530 | **3.** 2349 | **5.** 1945 |
| **2.** 2050 | **4.** 0315 | |

Solve the Story Problem

| | | |
|---|---|---|
| **1.** 6:00 a.m., 12:00 p.m., 6:00 p.m., and 12:00 a.m. | **2.** 101 °F, 103 °F | **4.** 1000 mg |
| | **3.** 165 lbs. | |

# Chapter 9: Putting It All Together

## Practice Exercise 9-1

**1.** List the eight steps needed to solve a story problem.

1. Read the questions

2. Read the story

3. Interpret what is being asked

4. Identify extraneous information

5. Identify and extract information needed to set up the equation

6. Set up the equation

7. Solve the equation

8. Solve the story problem

**2.** 3, 2, 5

**3.** 8, 24, 28, 36

**4.** $\frac{6}{7}$

**5.** 1. A letter can only be repeated **THREE** times.

2. If a letter is placed **BEFORE** another letter of **greater** value than **subtract** the smaller amount. **ONLY** subtract powers of 10.

3. If a letter is placed **AFTER** another letter of **greater** value than **add** the smaller amount.

**6.** 10

**7.** 81

**8.** 95

**9.** 18

**10.** LXXVII

**11.** D

**12.** XLV

## Practice Exercise 9-2

**1.** 26

**2.** 12

**3.** 108

**4.** 22

**5.** Multiplication

**6.** Addition

**7.** CXL

**8.** LXXXVIII

**9.** 59

**10.** 152

## Practice Exercise 9-3

**1.** 857

**2.** $\frac{9}{7}$

**3.** $1\frac{2}{7}$

**4.** Numerator

**5.** Mixed number

**6.** Multiplication, division

**7.** 1. $\frac{8}{9}$

   2. $\frac{3}{5}$

**8.** 1. $\frac{124}{15}$

   2. $\frac{23}{6}$

**9.** $\frac{V}{XLVII}$

**10.** 1. Proper fraction

   2. Improper fraction

   3. Mixed number

## Practice Exercise 9-4

1. 4365

2. $1\dfrac{7}{9}$

3. $\dfrac{2}{3}$

4. 852

5. $1\dfrac{1}{2}$

6. $I\dfrac{I}{II}$, or I ss

7. 1. 20

    2. 18

8. $\dfrac{2}{15}$

9. Invert

10. Common

## Practice Exercise 9-5

1. 8 is in the tens place

2. 4 is in the thousandths place

3. 6 is in the hundreds place

4. $\dfrac{VII}{XX}$, $\dfrac{7}{20}$, 0.35, 0.4

5. $4\dfrac{1}{6}$, 4.1667, 4.2

6. $\dfrac{10}{90}$, $\dfrac{1}{9}$, 0.111, 0.11

7. $\dfrac{45}{75}$, $\dfrac{9}{15}$, 0.6

8. $7\dfrac{75}{100}$, $7\dfrac{3}{4}$, $VII\dfrac{III}{IV}$

9. $2\dfrac{5}{10}$, $2\dfrac{1}{2}$, $II\dfrac{I}{II}$, or II ss

10. $4\dfrac{50}{1000}$, $4\dfrac{1}{20}$, $IV\dfrac{I}{XX}$

## Practice Exercise 9-6

1. 68.55 = 68.6

2. 1177.03 = 1177.0 = 1177

3. 261.578 = 261.58 = 261.6

4. 1268.406 = 1268.41 = 1268.4

5. 75.175 = 75.18 = 75.2

6. 2.580, 2.58, $\dfrac{258}{100}$, $2\dfrac{58}{100}$

7. 1.837, 1.84, $\dfrac{184}{100}$, $1\dfrac{84}{100}$, $1\dfrac{21}{25}$

8. 20.222, 20.22, $20\dfrac{22}{100}$, $20\dfrac{11}{50}$

9. 651.252, 651.25, $651\dfrac{25}{100}$, $651\dfrac{1}{4}$

10. 4.3, $\dfrac{43}{10}$, $4\dfrac{3}{10}$

## Practice Exercise 9-7

1. 475%

2. 87%

3. 3.97, $3\dfrac{97}{100}$

4. 1.75, $1\dfrac{75}{100}$, $1\dfrac{3}{4}$

5. 80 : 100, $\dfrac{80}{100}$, $\dfrac{4}{5}$, 80 : 100 :: 4 : 5

6. 15 : 45, $\dfrac{15}{45}$, $\dfrac{1}{3}$, 15 : 45 :: 1 : 3

7. $\dfrac{1}{3}$, $\dfrac{5}{15} = \dfrac{1}{3}$

8. $\dfrac{1}{8}$, $\dfrac{6}{48} = \dfrac{1}{8}$

9. ? = 2, $\dfrac{8}{12} = \dfrac{2}{3}$

10. ? = 18, $\dfrac{18}{81} = \dfrac{2}{9}$

## Practice Exercise 9-8

1. 6 tbsp.
2. 52.3 kg
3. 200 drops
4. 360 mL

5. 7.5 L
6. 250 mg
7. 0945 hours
8. 5:45 PM

9. °F − 32 ÷ 1.8 = °C
10. °C × 1.8 + 32 = °F

# Comprehensive Exam (Chapters 1 to 8)

1. F
2. F
3. T
4. F
5. T
6. F
7. T

8. F
9. T
10. T
11. eight
12. place holder
13. left
14. mixed number

15. metric system
16. 10
17. 8
18. 1400 hours
19. 15
20. divide

21. A term used in the metric system to measure mass.

22. A mathematical term to describe the answer to a division equation.

23. A mathematical term to describe the number "that is being divided."

24. The system of measurement used in the United States.

25. The sum of two or more numbers.

26. A mathematical term referring to two equal fractions or ratios.

27. The value of a number in multiples of 10, based on the digit's placement.

28. Any amount that is a part of 100.

29. A metric term used to describe volume.

30. A change from one system to another with the same or equal value.

31. 45.4
32. 5.9
33. $1\frac{23}{60}$
34. $\frac{65}{141}$
35. 7 r 47
36. 152.6 F°
37. 50 mL
38. 5 oz.
39. 139.5

40. $14\frac{21}{40}$
41. $\frac{7}{11}$ (lowest terms)
42. 3465
43. 1900 hours
44. $\frac{3}{10} = \frac{15}{? = 50}$
45. 35000 mg
46. 30.6 °C
47. XXXI = 31
48. 518.6

49. 8 r 15
50. 0.7
51. $\frac{16}{25}$
52. $12\frac{4}{15}$
53. 536
54. 0.6
55. 33938.1
56. 23 L
57. 64.5 kg

**58.** $11\frac{23}{32}$

**59.** 11:00 p.m.

**60.** 536

**61.** 33%

**62.** VIII.II = 8.2

**63.** 237.6 lbs.

**64.** 372 : 103

**65.** $\frac{71}{103} = \frac{?}{100}$, 68.93%

**66.** $\frac{20}{103} = \frac{?}{100}$, 19.42%

**67.** $\frac{71}{103} + \frac{20}{103} = \frac{91}{103}$, $\frac{91}{103} = \frac{?}{100}$, 88.35%

**68.** Yes

**69.** 10

**70.** $2575.00

# Glossary of Key Terms

**Addition**  A mathematical operation that represents the total or sum of two or more objects or numbers. Addition is represented in a math equation with a "plus sign" (+).

**Centi**  A prefix used in the metric system to represent one hundredth.

**Common Denominator**  The number quantity by which all denominators in a set of fractions may be divided evenly. Used in adding and subtracting fractions.

**Conversion**  A change from one system to another with the same or equal value.

**Cross Multiplication**  A mathematical method in which a numerator of a fraction is multiplied by the denominator of another fraction.

**Decimals**  Any number of parts of a whole number separated using a decimal point.

**Decrease**  The act of taking one or more numbers or objects away from a larger amount of numbers or objects.

**Denominator**  A mathematical term used to identify and describe the bottom number of a fraction. The *total of all parts*, as represented in a fraction.

**Difference**  A mathematical term to describe the answer to a subtraction equation.

**Dividend**  A mathematical term to describe the number "*that is being divided.*"

**Division**  A mathematical operation that separates the entire value of a number into multiple smaller-value parts. Division is represented in a math equation with a "division sign" (÷) or (/).

**Divisor**  A mathematical term to describe the number "*divided by.*"

**Equation**  A mathematical expression that contains two or more numbers, a mathematical calculation or action and a conclusion or answer.

**Fraction**  Any number of parts of a whole number or object.

**Gram**  A term used in the metric system to measure mass.

**Household System**  The system of measurement used in the United States.

**Improper Fraction**  A mathematical term used to identify and describe a fraction that has a larger number as the numerator (top number) and a smaller number as the denominator (bottom number).

**Increase**  The act of adding one or more numbers to a given number.

**Invert**  To turn upside down.

**Kilo**  A prefix used in the metric system to represent one thousand.

**Liter**  A metric term used to describe volume.

**Lowest Terms**  The action of reducing (dividing) a larger fraction to its lowest possible term or represented value.

**Metric System**  A system of measurement based on multiples of 10 used in the medical industry and most countries outside the United States.

**Micro**  A prefix used in the metric system to represent one millionth.

**Milli**  A prefix used in the metric system to represent one thousandth.

**Mixed Numbers**  A mathematical expression using a whole number and a fraction, often converted from an improper fraction.

**Multiplication**  A mathematical operation that repeats a number's value multiple times. Multiplication is represented in a math equation with a "multiplication sign" ($\times$).

**Numerator**  A mathematical term used to identify and describe the top number of fraction. The amount of parts you *have*, as represented in a fraction.

**Percent**  Any amount that is a part of 100.

**Place Holder**  A digit that has no value and is used to assist in lining numbers up in columns in a mathematical equation, is always a zero (0).

**Place Value**  The value of a number in multiples of 10, based on the digit's placement.

**Product**  A mathematical term to describe the answer to a multiplication equation.

**Proper Fraction**  A mathematical term used to identify and describe a fraction that has a smaller number as the numerator (top number) and a larger number as the denominator (bottom number). Often reduced to lowest terms.

**Proportion**  A mathematical term referring to two equal fractions or ratios.

**Quotient**  A mathematical term to describe the answer to a division equation.

**Ratio**  A mathematical statement of how two numbers compare. How much of one item or number as compared to another item or number.

**Reciprocal**  A mathematical term to describe an inverted fraction.

**Rounding**  Either increasing or decreasing a number to the next digit based on number place value.

**Simplify**  A mathematical term used to express the action of reducing fractions to lowest terms.

**Subtraction**  A mathematical operation that represents the removal or taking away of an object or number from a larger amount. Subtraction is represented in a math equation with a "minus sign" (–).

**Sum**  A mathematical term to describe the answer to an addition equation.

**Total**  The sum of two or more numbers or objects.

**Unit of Measurement**  A division of any quantity that represents an accepted standard of measurement.

# Index